LET IT GO

Breathe Yourself Calm

REBECCA DENNIS

CONTENTS

INTRODUCTION

LET IT GO

Breathe Yourself Calm

REBECCA DENNIS

if we've never heard the science, that how we breathe and how we feel are intrinsically linked.

The practice of breathwork is, simply put, breathing exercises that allow you to change and manipulate the rhythm, depth and rate of your breath with intention and purpose to improve your physical, mental and emotional performance. Optimum breathing plays a pivotal role in your overall health and in the proper functioning of your immune and nervous systems. Using your breath to its full potential can help strengthen your lungs and pulmonary system while reducing anxiety and stress. By learning to breathe well you limit your risk of burning out and naturally defend your immune system.

Breathwork has become a buzzword, not only in the wellness world but in corporate life and education too. But, really understanding and learning the basics of better breathing means that instead of going somewhere to be 'fixed', you can use your body's natural abilities to help yourself. Constant tension in the body can lead to anxious thought patterns, bad digestion, a weaker immune system, and increased acidity and inflammation – it's all connected. Science is now catching up with what the sages and yogis have been saying for thousands of years: our emotions and breathing are fundamentally linked.

BREATHE YOURSELF BETTER

Breathing exercises are proven to have lasting effects on both your physical and mental health, providing a method you can use every day to help navigate your way through life. The breath is a barometer to your inner state of being. I have seen first-hand the power that better breathing can have to help us face, recover and heal from trauma, pain and fear.

As I write this book, we are collectively going through a mass trauma. In these times we are reminded that the only certainty is that nothing is ever certain. While the world is spinning and we are all trying to adapt and find some sort of stability, there is one thing that is always constant – and that is our breath.

Breathing is the only autonomic system in the body that you can learn to control to change your sense of wellbeing and anchor your mind. Most of us hold physical, mental and emotional tension in our bodies which can impact our health. Although we cannot change or control everything around us, we can control our response and how it affects our physiology. Breathing exercises help you release tension and unprocessed trauma, break unhealthy patterns and coping mechanisms and quieten the chatter in your mind. Indeed, this profound power we all possess can be used every day to change our breathing patterns, thereby altering our nervous system and state of mind.

'We can change how we
react, act and feel by simply
changing the rhythms of
our breath.'

You may have heard how sages and experts are able to
reach states of bliss and enlightenment by using their breath
as a superpower after years of dedication and training but
here's a newsflash: you don't have to be wealthy, spiritual or
a guru to feel the benefit of breathing exercises. One breath
at a time, you can move towards reaching goals that may
have felt unattainable with a deeper understanding of your
breath, bringing tangible results that do not require years of
rigorous practice, right now.

'Life is 10% what happens
to us and 90% how we
breathe through it.'

Embrace your breath

Every day you have a choice to take your breath for
granted or to fully embrace and feel everything that life
gives you. All thoughts, experiences and feelings directly

stimulate your physiology and influence how you breathe. Breathing exercises can create a pause between stimulus and response, helping you to remain grounded and process life events. The key is creating space between stressful moments to recalibrate and reset rather than staying wired. Breathing is free, and not particularly hard, yet many of us hold or limit our breath subconsciously to keep life at bay.

You'll know you have understood the art of breathwork when the way you respond to your circumstances changes, even if the circumstances themselves have not. One of the most courageous decisions you can ever make is to choose to live in the now, and that is an active process. Conscious breathing is a critical tool that can ground you in the present, allowing you to move through life in a healthy way. Rather than burying your feelings or trying to erase a memory, you can learn to fully feel and accept all your experiences and work with them rather than against them.

When you change the way you breathe, you change something fundamental in your whole physiology. You can change your state from feeling anxious to calm, scattered to focused, even from tired to more energised. In short, you can rewire your nervous system and supercharge your mind! Breathwork provides you with a life-long set of tools to use every day to help navigate your way through life, and even transform it if you want to.

HOW TO USE THIS BOOK

This book is the culmination of over 20 years of my work in breath- and body-based therapy. I've worked with thousands of people each with their own unique needs, including autoimmune disease, chronic obstructive pulmonary disease (COPD), depression, cancer and addiction, and my clients include veterans, teachers, NHS staff, boxers, celebrities, opera singers, actors, entrepreneurs, high-flying city workers, musicians, yogis and elite athletes. Over the last decade, my mission has been to make breathwork accessible to as many people as possible and to all ages – from workplaces to schools to care homes and hospitals. During the recent coronavirus pandemic, NHS workers, teachers and people working on the front line have used my techniques to help them manage daily stress and trauma.

We are all wired differently. There is no 'one size fits all' philosophy here – what calms one person in one situation may not work for someone else. This book will show how you can incorporate different simple breathing exercises into all areas of everyday life and find the ones that work best for you. You'll find an abundance of effective breathing techniques, combined with other methods such as self-acupressure; mindset positivity; body-based therapy; and movement and sound to empower, inspire and energise. I encourage you to incorporate these methods into your life in simple steps that you can build on as you go deeper. But if you are just starting out and getting to grips with breathwork, then focus on the .

breathing exercises for now – they are powerful enough on their own.

Each chapter has its own 'remedy bag' of breathing exercises and techniques to try. Alongside other tips to support and heal the body in a natural way, these remedies are prescribed to aid different situations and strengthen your body's natural defences, from dealing with stress to boosting energy, from coping with trauma and grief to getting a restorative night's sleep. Not all categories will be relevant to you the first time you read this book, but they all relate to the total human experience. You can use these exercises not just to help yourself but also as a remedy to share with others in your life who may need support now or in the future.

I've also included a section for families because breathwork really is for all ages – we teach our young to walk and talk yet how to use the breath is forgotten. With rising rates in anxiety in young people these are empowering tools for life. The methods I've included are both modern and ancient – some have been used for over thousands of years – this is seriously tried-and-tested self-help!

This book works on two levels: for those who want to dive in and read the whole thing in one sitting but also as a loyal companion to dip into at your bedside, on the move or before a presentation, whenever you're in need of breathing space.

You've been breathing all your life, so you may assume that you will be 'good at' breathing exercises and perhaps at times this book might challenge you, bringing frustration if exercises don't always come easily. Approach the exercises with curiosity, especially if you notice resistance. Resistance can be a flag that you are trying to avoid spending time with yourself. It is a choice to practise letting go. No one else can do that for you. The idea of this responsibility can feel overwhelming and may trigger self-doubt. A lack of belief in your own power to make changes can stop you in your tracks but you are more powerful than you realise.

There's a myriad of advice on building resilience for overwhelm and anxiety but a lot of it involves major lifestyle changes or upgrades that feel inaccessible, impossible, expensive or just unlikely. This book focuses on helping you to learn how to let go without needing equipment or accessories, without adding to your to-do list or making radical changes to your schedule. It is your personal support system, offering simple techniques that will work for you in any situation.

Learning to control and understand your breath can be the most profound and transformational relationship you will ever have. Breathwork does not ask for perfection. You do not need to worry whether you're 'doing it right'. The overthinking part of our minds can often put us off our tracks; it uses all of its power to draw us away from being present with this magical gift we were born with. Even on days when it feels like nothing has shifted, there are always little evolutions happening in your nervous system and the corners of your mindset. There are times when you may feel challenged, so please go easy on yourself, be open to how the exercises might expand what you know and enable entirely new ways to experience the environment around you.

I want to encourage you to trust and explore your own inner compass, to use your breath and be flexible and experimental with which methods suit you. Many of us have mastered how to live in survival mode but that is no way to travel through life. It's time for a breath revolution! Let's get started . . .

UNDERSTANDING
YOUR BREATH

You've been breathing all your life and it's probably something you take for granted because you don't have to think about it. In the same way that you blink, your heart beats and your digestive system functions, your breath is automatic. But unlike other natural functions, you can also actively use your breath to help with any task at hand, whether it's physical performance – such as diving, running or cycling – or mental focus, to physically heal yourself or to deepen your awareness.

You could liken it to when you first learn to swim or walk; it takes a tremendous amount of concentration to begin with but eventually it becomes second nature. When you first begin to develop an awareness of your breath it takes conscious effort and practice, but in time you'll find it easier and it will always be there for you when you need it.

'The way you breathe is indicative of how you feel about life; it's no exaggeration to say it's essential to your mental and physical wellbeing.'

GOOD BREATHING VS DYSFUNCTIONAL BREATHING

Despite the recent explosion of interest in wellness and an increasing appreciation of how important our health is, very few people are aware of the detrimental effects that improper breathing can have on their wellbeing. While most of us know instinctively how to breathe to survive, we aren't all taught how to breathe to thrive.

It is a common belief that we breathe with our lungs alone, but the work of breathing is done by the whole body. The lungs play a passive role in the respiratory process. Their expansion is produced by an enlargement, mostly downwards, of the thoracic cavity and they collapse when that cavity is reduced. Good breathing involves the head, neck, thorax, pelvis and abdomen muscles, while chronic tension in any part of the body interferes with the natural respiratory movements.

Breathing is a rhythmic activity. At rest an average person takes 12–17 breaths a minute. The rate is higher when you are excited, and in infants, and lower when you're asleep and in those who are depressed. The depth of the respiratory wave also varies with emotional states. Breathing becomes shallow when you are frightened or anxious. It deepens with relaxation, pleasure and sleep. But above all, it is the quality of the respiratory movements that determines whether breathing is pleasurable or not. With each breath a wave ascends and descends through the body. The respiratory wave (or inhale) begins deep in the abdomen with a backwards movement of the pelvis. This allows the belly to expand outwards. The wave then moves upwards as the rest of the body expands. The expiration wave (or exhale) begins in the upper part of the body and moves downwards: the chest and abdomen contract, and the pelvis rocks forwards.

A guide to some common dysfunctional breathing patterns

Chest breathing – The movement of the breath is more in the upper chest. The shoulders rise on the inhale and there is a tendency to overuse secondary breathing muscles and ones you do not need for breathing in the shoulders and neck. This can cause tension in the upper back and shoulders. There can be a lot of tension in the diaphragm as well and little movement in the belly area when breathing. This is the most common pattern I come across and it forms over time from holding the belly in to look thinner and as a response to stress. More extreme chest breathing patterns with the chest aggressively puffing out on the inhale with no movement in the belly are noticeable in people who work out obsessively or those with high levels of anxiety.

Belly breathing – The movement of the breath is seen mostly in the belly. The chest and shoulders are still with not much movement in the ribcage. The belly expands on the inhale and contracts on the exhale. The upper back can often feel tense with a posture looking like there is a layer of armour or a shell of protection. As the intercostal muscles (muscles in between the ribs) are not being used as much, this can restrict the movement of the diaphragm, reducing lung capacity. You can feel more grounded and present when breathing in the belly but also carry emotional armour around the chest area protecting the heart.

Shallow breathing – The movement of the breath is not as visible. We become shallow breathers during periods of stress, when we are depressed, when we've not had much sleep, have had a bad day at work or the kids are playing up. Often if people are in pain, they will shallow breathe to avoid feeling that pain. Shallow breathing results in lower amounts of lymphocyte, a type of white blood cell that helps to defend the body from invading organisms, and lowers the amount of proteins that signal other immune cells. The body is then more susceptible to contracting acute illnesses, aggravating pre-existing medical conditions and prolonging healing times. Shallow breathing can be a coping mechanism to avoid panic attacks and cause dry mouth and fatigue.

Frozen breath – Frozen breathing, as described by breathing expert Donna Fahri, is when the entire outer layer of the body contracts and suppresses the rising movement of the breath. When you breathe freely, the inner and outer body move with one another. In frozen breathing, the outer container remains rigid. The root of this breathing pattern can be fear of not being good enough, not becoming 'someone', or early deep-rooted trauma.

Reverse breathing – This is not so common and will take regular practice and commitment to correct. An open breath should show the belly expanding on the inhale. However, with reverse breathing the breath starts in the upper chest and pulls the abdomen towards the spine. This means that the stomach muscles are contracted most of the time and both the inhale and exhale can feel tight and controlled. By lying on the floor and breathing into the ground for a few minutes every day you can retrain the pattern over time. This breathing pattern can be caused by many things from spinal issues to early trauma.

Breath holding – This is another common breathing pattern when you are multitasking – texting and emailing and realising you haven't actually taken a breath. It is also a subconscious behaviour to want to metaphorically hide away. If the diaphragm is restricted, the breath is shallow and confined to the chest. This overstimulates the sympathetic nervous system, which controls the body's fight-or-flight response, and results in the physiological symptoms of stress and feelings of anxiety. It also tends to keep you locked into your worries and anxious thoughts.

By first becoming aware you are a breath holder, you are on the path to correcting it and reminding yourself to breathe.

There are other patterns such as over-breathing and cases where people are overusing their lower back muscles to breathe. Breathing feels like an effort and they subconsciously feel they have to work hard at everything, finding it hard to let go of control and be in the flow. There are many more intricate patterns and each one tells a story. The more you practise breathing well, the more you let go of any restricted breathing patterns and old habits.

ARE YOU A BELLY BREATHER
OR A CHEST BREATHER?

This simple exercise can help you begin to understand your breathing pattern.

o Sitting up keep your spine straight. Relax your shoulders, try not to hunch them. Close your eyes.

o Take a deep inhale through your nose and exhale through your nose.

o Repeat 2–3 times.

o Now, place one hand on your belly and the other hand on your chest. Breathe in through your nose and out through your nose. Notice where you can feel the breath more. Can you feel it more in your chest or can you feel it more in your belly? Or can you feel it equally in both? Wherever you can feel it more indicates your dominant breathing pattern.

FINDING YOUR WAY TO A HEALTHY BREATH

These are some easy first steps to help correct your breath pattern and achieve an open, healthy breath.

Start in the belly – By inhaling into the belly, the abdomen is pushed outwards causing the diaphragm to extend downwards, opening up the lower part of your lungs. This is extremely beneficial since it is the area with the highest density of alveoli – the small air sacks that transfer oxygen into your bloodstream.

Come up into the midsection – Once your breath is fully in the abdomen, the breath wave moves across the diaphragm and up to the ribcage. It is within the diaphragm area that most restrictions are found. Known as the fear belt, this part of your body carries most of your emotional trauma and muscular tension from fight-or-flight responses.

Move into the chest area – Once across the diaphragm, the breath travels up the chest and across the heart. The heart area is the second area that is often congested, mostly with tight muscular responses from repressed emotions. We hold on to a lot of tension in the shoulders and upper chest. Often, when you feel stressed or are finding it hard to let go, these areas can feel constricted and can lead to panic attacks and anxiety.

The throat area – Once past the heart area, the breath wave peaks into the upper chest and throat. It is at the top of the breath wave that the secondary breathing muscles (sternocleidomastoid, trapezius and pectoralis minor) come into play. These secondary muscles provide balance and stability to your breathing system but being much lighter than the primary muscles, they also tire more rapidly. When working with the throat area, you may have some blockages around communication and expression. Another key place for holding tension is the jaw, where repressed emotions of anger or grief can manifest in teeth grinding.

How can you breathe better?

We are all wired differently – from our genetics, to our DNA, endocrine systems and our breathing patterns. Different exercises will work for different people, but there are basic steps that we can all take to improve our breathing and wellbeing:

– understanding a healthy breathing pattern and using your breath to its full capacity.

– quietening and decluttering your mind so you can make choices as opposed to being reactive.

– understanding your emotions and how your subconscious can prevent you from being your best self.

To harness the power of your breath you don't need to learn new tricks, you just need to remember how you used to breathe. If you want to find a true breath guru, take a look at a sleeping baby. When we are babies and toddlers, our breath is full and flowing with no tension in the belly, chest, back or diaphragm. And yet the majority of teenagers and adults lose their natural ability to breathe fully and use as little as a third of their respiratory systems.

As babies and toddlers, we felt no inhibitions and had no awareness of feelings of fear, shame, guilt or embarrassment. We expressed exactly how we felt and were completely present. Our minds were not flitting all over the place and we were not trying to control our emotions or feelings by holding our breath or breathing shallowly to hide or not be heard.

Between the ages of three and seven, we begin to develop emotionally, becoming more aware of our surroundings, culture, peer groups and authority in the home and at school. In short, we become conditioned through being instructed – told to calm down, be quiet or brave. All these instructions create boundaries and obstacles when we are feeling emotions such as anger, embarrassment, frustration, sadness, guilt, joy, or even if we are trying to stop ourselves from laughing. Dysfunctional breathing comes from learned behaviour as well – boys mirroring men puffing out their chests to look strong, children being told to tuck their tummies in and keep their spines straight in gymnastics and dance classes. As a result of these moments, when you hold your breath or control your breathing, the muscles within your respiratory system contract and store these memories in your tissues and fascia. Your body is like a biological recording of your past, holding on to all these stories.

Our breathing patterns mirror our life patterns, yet some of these established patterns are not serving us well. When you begin to clear these restricted breathing patterns, you can open and expand your breath and live life more freely. Like any practice, the most challenging part of breathwork is just sitting down to do it. Starting small and simple is key, and if you practise every day it will soon become a way of life.

BREATH AWARENESS

Every day you have a choice whether to take your breath for granted or to breathe fully, and to feel and embrace everything that life offers. Start with this exercise to help you to become aware of your breath and notice how you are breathing right now. This allows you to quieten the thoughts in your head and connect to the feelings in your body.

As you read this . . .

o Notice how your breath moves in your body. Focus on and observe your breath. Let your mind follow the flow of your breath . . . Observe, feel, witness your breath coming and going . . .

o How do you feel right now? Whether it's positive or negative, without judging or controlling, just accept those feelings, noticing your breath and how you feel . . .

o Focusing on your breath is the most effective way to check in on how you really feel, so ask yourself: Am I tired? Am I happy? Am I anxious? Am I relaxed? Is my mind full? Am I overthinking? Am I focused?

o Are you carrying any tension? Where does it feel tight? Where does it feel freer? Become aware of physical sensations, notice the contact of your feet on the ground, your sitting bones on the chair or floor, notice your spine and the length of your spine – is it straight? Are you hunching?

○ Simply notice your breath and become more conscious of the inhale and exhale. Focus on bringing in more breath in a relaxed, flowing motion. Slowly breathing in through your nose and slowly breathing out through your nose. Just notice how that feels.

○ As you breathe in and out, pay attention to whether your jaw is relaxed or if you are slightly clenching it. Relax your jaw, allow space between the top and bottom jaws and drop your shoulders. Just by becoming aware of your breath, you can start to feel truly present and conscious of how you feel.

○ Take slow, gentle breaths, Now inhale for as long as you can and exhale for as long as you can. Bringing full awareness to your breath moves you from 'doing' to 'being'.

○ Bring the movement of your breath down into your lower abdominals. See if you can move the belly as you breathe in and out. This is where you start to consciously breathe with intention.

○ Expand your breath into your lower belly as you inhale and contract as you exhale. As you inhale your belly expands and as you exhale the belly contracts.

○ Now breathe in for a count of three and breathe out for a count of three. Simple, easy breaths, in through the nose and out through the nose with no force, pushing or trying to control the breath. Exhale one, two, three.

○ Keep practising this for a few more breaths, going at your own count and pace. Remain aware of your breath, observing how the inhale and exhale feel. Is it easier to inhale than to exhale or the other way round? Or do both feel the same?

Making friends with your diaphragm

As babies and toddlers, we naturally breathe deeply from the diaphragm and one of the first steps towards a healthy breath is practising diaphragmatic breathing. This is not about learning new tricks, it is about remembering how you used to breathe. Although this can be easy to achieve, it takes repetition for the muscles to remember and requires letting go of old patterns for it to become automatic. You can hold tension in the diaphragm, especially when you are controlling pain or emotions. You need to work with your primary breathing muscles – the lower abdominal muscles and intercostal muscles – to achieve a good diaphragmatic breath.

When teaching breathwork, I begin with the diaphragm as most are tight which doesn't necessarily mean strong. In Chinese medicine the diaphragm is described as the gateway between the upper and lower body, regulating the flow of energy throughout the body. Our ability to breathe well diaphragmatically is hindered by stress, lack of muscle strength and of awareness. The diaphragm also works with other respiratory muscles, so if the movement is restricted it can create tension in the jaw, psoas muscle and hips (see pages 29–39 for exercises to help open these areas).

When your fight-or-flight response is frequently triggered, you default to chest breathing and the breath can feel jerky, rapid, irregular or shallow. If this becomes habitual, these muscles become overused and the breath becomes restricted to the chest. Since the blood capillaries are more generously distributed in the lower lungs, upper chest breathing results in a less efficient oxygen exchange than deep diaphragmatic breathing.

Your diaphragm is a dome-shaped sheet of tonic muscle and tendon which plays a vital role in the breathing process. As you breathe in, you should feel the belly expand slightly as the dome contracts and compresses the abdominal space and as you breathe out, both the ribcage and belly should contract. Take a moment to visualise where the diaphragm is in your body. The organs above the diaphragm need to be connected and in communication with the organs below it, so there are openings for blood vessels and nerves.

The breath is the bridge linking your mind and body. The practice of conscious diaphragmatic breathing helps to stimulate your parasympathetic nervous system (PNS), which allows your body to rest and digest, slow the heart rate, lower blood pressure and respiratory rate and divert blood supply towards the digestive and reproductive systems. When the PNS is active, the sympathetic nervous system (SNS) which raises heart rate, blood pressure and respiratory rate, diverting blood to the brain and skeletal muscle in readiness for fight-or-flight, becomes less active. By deactivating or overriding your SNS, you can interrupt the vicious cycle of adrenaline and cortisol which contribute to chronic stress and can predispose you to anxiety and panic attacks.

The expansion and contraction of the diaphragm when you breathe can stimulate your lymphatic system and

27

'massage' your internal organs. The lymphatic system
works with the immune system to help the body
remove internal toxins, so something as simple as
breathing well can increase your body's natural
detoxification process.

DEEP DIAPHRAGMATIC BREATHING

You can do this exercise sitting up anywhere – at your desk, on the train or at home on the sofa. This exercise helps to bring awareness to your breathing and ground and focus your attention. Practise it as many times as you like; think of it as a mini workout for the respiratory system.

- Place your hands on your belly so you can feel your breath expanding and moving through your body. Relax your jaw, face and shoulders. When you breathe in, the diaphragm contracts and flattens downwards, creating a vacuum that draws in air. When you exhale, the diaphragm returns to its dome shape, pushing air out of your body.

- Keep your spine long, feel your sitting bones on your seat and your feet flat on the ground. Hold your head in a neutral position as if there is a thread through the top of your head, holding it up towards the sky. Relax your throat and jaw.

- Breathe in slowly through your nose. Let the air flow as you inhale and expand your belly – expanding your sides and lower ribs, diaphragm, back and lower back. Allow a slow, gentle inhale to expand your belly. Exhale with a gentle sigh through your nose or mouth and feel the belly contract.

- Place your hands around your lower ribcage as if you are giving yourself a hug and breath into this space.

Expand your belly as you inhale and contract as you exhale. Keep your shoulders and jaw relaxed.

o Repeat 10–20 times and notice how you feel. Present, grounded, sleepy, relaxed?

Tip: If you are finding it hard to bring the breath down into the belly, lie face down on the floor and breathe into the ground so you can feel your belly pushing on the ground as you inhale and letting go as you exhale. See if you can then get the breath movement to come down into the pelvis. Make a little pillow for your head with your hands and practise this for a few minutes every day. This will eventually help to bring the breath movement lower down and activate these primary breathing muscles.

The three diaphragms

Most of us are aware of the diaphragm that separates
the thoracic and abdominal cavities, however there
are two other diaphragms that play a vital role in allowing
this central diaphragm to work effectively: the pelvic and
vocal diaphragms. (There are more diaphragms in the
respiratory system, but in this book I will concentrate on
these main three.)

The pelvic diaphragm lies at the base of the pelvis and the
vocal diaphragm is situated in the upper part of the air
passage between the trachea and base of the tongue.
When the abdomen is chronically tight, the pelvic
diaphragm is held in a state of contraction and you may

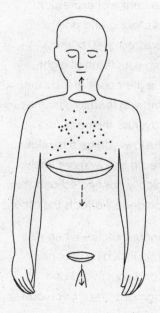
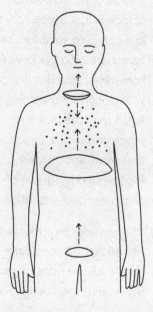

also experience tightness in the hips. Holding tension in your pelvic and vocal diaphragms affects the ability of the main diaphragm to move freely up and down. By bringing your awareness to these three diaphragms and helping to release chronic tension, you can free your breath and increase your lung capacity. Imagine the diaphragms as doors that blow open or shut depending on where your energy is moving.

The jaw

When teaching the foundations of breathwork and release points, the jaw is one of the starting points. The jaw muscles are some of the first muscles we instinctively use as babies to suckle, express and communicate. Within these muscles is years of stored memory. It is the centre of expression, or lack of it. A chronically tight or clicking and painful jaw can be a symptom of unexpressed grief, or stress from clenching the jaw or grinding your teeth at night. Sometimes your breathing can be the cause of the issue. With abnormal breathing patterns, you tend to alter the function of the diaphragm and overuse the neck and shoulder muscles. By softening the jaw, you help to relax the diaphragm, allowing your breath to flow more freely. The jaw and pelvis are physiologically connected and the alignment and relaxation of each deeply affects the other.

The masseter (jaw muscle) is a signal muscle – when your jaw relaxes other muscles relax too, including your neck, forehead, the base of your skull and your throat and shoulders. When using a diaphragmatic breath, you can learn to relax the jaw at the same time. By relaxing the jaw you are helping the largest muscle in your body to relax too.

As you're breathing right now, relax your jaw, teeth slightly apart. Breathe in through your nose and out through your nose, allow the tip of your tongue to rest on the palate of your mouth and allow the bottom jaw to relax.

JAW RELEASE

Gentle acupressure while breathing through the mouth is a really great way to release tension from the jaw.

o Use your second and third fingers to gently massage the muscle that sits between the meeting of the top and bottom jaw. You can yawn or sigh or use exaggerated mouth movements to help release this area more deeply.

o With clean hands and clipped fingernails, massage the inside of your mouth and particularly the large muscles at the back that are responsible for opening and closing the jaw. You will be amazed how hard these muscles can feel, almost like bones. Simply holding gentle pressure there can start to release some of the muscle tension.

Hip flexors and psoas muscle

I often refer to the hips as the drawer we throw items in when we don't know where else to put them, or can't quite let them go yet. Just as you clench the jaw, the same action unconsciously happens in your hips. Each time you hold back emotion, feel threatened or have a stress reaction, you physically respond by tensing in this area or by metaphorically drawing yourself in or running away to protect yourself. The natural response to stress is to use your hips to take flight, kick out, fight or recoil into a foetal position to protect your core. These contractions not only store muscular tension but also deep emotion felt at that time. When the jaw or hips are tight, these muscles are also more restricted.

The psoas is a deep-set core muscle otherwise known as the muscle of the soul. Originating from the lumbar vertebrae, it forms a strip of muscle along each side of the spine. Since the psoas is closely linked to your fight-or-flight mechanism, fear can be over-represented in those with constricted psoas. Trauma can lead to back, hip and knee issues as well as digestive and dysfunctional breathing. The psoas connects the upper body to the lower body, linking the breath to movement, feelings and healing. By restoring balance to your psoas muscles using your breath, you can release any pent-up tension, improving your physical and mental wellbeing. Practising stretching and disciplines such as qigong or gentle yoga can help the body to release and uncoil using co-ordinated movement, breathing and meditation. Lunges, pigeon pose and side bends are all good beginner poses to work with when releasing tension and old trauma.

Horizontal breathing vs vertical breathing

The difference between these two ways of breathing is that the first is the way we were designed to breathe and the other is how we've learned to breathe over time. Take a deep breath right now and notice how your breath moves. We accumulate a lot of tension in the shoulders by repeatedly using the shoulder, chest and neck muscles to move with the breath. You may find that when you take a deep breath in your shoulders rise up towards your ears and the breath puffs out your chest with not much movement in the belly area. You may feel movement in the mid-section but a tightness in your chest and less movement in the lower abdominals. This is known as clavicular or vertical breathing. If you suffer from shoulder and neck pain, then vertical breathing is likely contributing to your discomfort. Vertical breathing puts unnecessary strain on the shoulders and neck muscles from overuse. Paired with today's more sedentary lifestyles, it is not a good combination.

Rather than your breath rising up and down, visualise and feel your breath moving in and out, expanding your belly, lower back and ribcage on the inhale and contracting as you exhale. I see a lot of people whose breath is moving vertically up and down and I would like to encourage and practise a more expansive horizontal breath – think of your breath expanding in and out like an accordion or bellows for a fire.

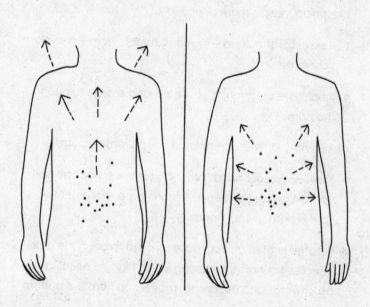

EXPAND YOUR BREATH

You can do this exercise anywhere to develop a better connection to your diaphragm and use this primary breathing muscle more effectively.

o Relax your shoulders – try not to hunch them – and close your eyes.

o Inhale deeply through your nose and exhale through the nose.

o Repeat 2–3 times, breathing in and breathing out.

o Now, wrap your hands around your lower ribcage as if you are giving yourself a hug. Bring the movement of your breath to your hands.

o Breathe in through your nose and out through the nose. Visualise your breath moving into a triangle pointing downwards and the breath moving up from the bottom point of the triangle.

o Notice where you can feel your breath and visualise it expanding in and out as opposed to up and down. Feel your breath moving your belly and ribcage as you keep your shoulders relaxed and your breath expansive.

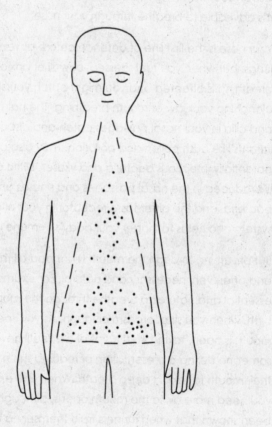

Nose breathing vs mouth breathing

I often get asked if it's better to breathe through the nose or the mouth. Mouth breathing can be used for more advanced breathing techniques, but in everyday life it's advisable to breathe through your nose.

Your nose is the first line of defence before air reaches your lungs, but when you feel stressed, unwell or anxious, your breathing is affected and you might catch yourself sighing, clenching your jaw or mouth breathing. The hairs, mucus and cilia in your nasal passages catch and dispose of irritants like dust, pollen and pollution. They also catch potentially infectious bacteria and viruses. Nitric oxide is produced in the nasal passages and sinuses and can kill bacteria, and the bitter taste receptor in your olfactory system also helps to trigger your body's immune response.

But breathing through the mouth is not bad all the time and often very necessary and natural. For example, it's essential and natural to breathe through the mouth during birth, when you sing, orgasm or laugh. As you speak, your mouth is open, taking in little sips of air. You'll never see someone during a presentation or reading the news close their mouth to take a deep breath. When you exercise, you need more air so the mouth opens, although it has been shown that when runners train themselves to breath only through their noses, it can increase their stamina and reduce fatigue.

I teach some exercises with the mouth open and some breathing through the nose. There is ongoing research in this area. If people want to breathe deeper or use the breath for therapeutic work, they often breathe through the mouth and, despite some claims that this stimulates the fight-or-flight response, when using mouth breathing techniques with intention, people can go into a very deep state of relaxation. The more you play with and explore breathing exercises, the more you become attuned to what techniques work for you.

HOW TO BREATHE WELL – FROM WAKE-UP TO BEDTIME

Conscious breathing is the basic foundation of breathing well. It can help you to develop an intimate relationship with your breath, so you can sense when it feels right or if it feels jerky, rapid and restricted, if it's more difficult to inhale or exhale, or both. You can bring back clarity and calm by intentionally manipulating the rate, depth, rhythm and pattern of your breath to send information to your limbic system, the part of the brain involved in behavioural and emotional responses.

These exercises are intended to help you connect with and use your breath throughout the day, to improve how you feel from the moment you wake up to winding down to sleep at night. (For specific exercises to help you get a restful night's sleep, see the chapter on Sleep, pages 204–209.)

WAKE UP AND GROUND

I use this exercise regularly to relax the muscles, calm the mind, promote circulation and create a sense of peace. It's an effective way to ground and check how you are feeling at the start of the day, prompting mental stillness while encouraging a deeper, more mindful breath. This exercise can be done sitting or lying down in bed to wake yourself up and feel more alert. You can also practise it at work or while studying to recharge and reboot your energy.

As it gets easier to sit for longer, add on a few rounds and begin to build a broader and more expansive breath. Notice where you feel more space, more length and more strength, and acknowledge where you feel more energy and alertness.

o Sit comfortably in an upright position (or lie down) and close your eyes.

o Draw a slow, long inhale through both nostrils for as long as is comfortable.

o Relax your shoulders and encourage the movement of your breath to be in your lower abdominals and ribcage. Soften your jaw.

o Hold the breath for as long as is comfortable – at no point should this feel difficult. Consciously rest your jaw, throat, neck, shoulders, diaphragm and abdominal muscles. The more relaxed you are, the easier it will be to hold the breath for longer.

o Exhale through both nostrils for as long as is comfortable.

o Repeat five rounds of this exercise and then pause and
   observe how you feel.

Tips: The inhale and exhale don't need to be a particular
length, nor do you need to observe any ratio between the
inhale and exhale. Make sure that the inhale and exhale
are deep and full and practised without struggle.

DAILY BREATH PRACTICE

This simple exercise will help you let go of tension while regulating the nervous system and reminding your body how you used to breathe before you became conditioned to restrict your breath. Practise this every day – in bed, on the way to work, in the shower. Some days you might notice you have more tension in the jaw or the shoulders, or your chest or just below the diaphragm.

o Breathe in through your nose for a count of six and breathe out through your nose for a count of six. Relax your jaw and shoulders and find a rhythm that is comfortable for you. By breathing this way, you are telling your brain: 'I am safe and relaxed'.

o Allow your breath to be relaxed and steady without trying to force it. If six counts feels too long, begin with three and then move to four. Be patient and don't push or force the breath.

o Just notice your breath, bringing all your awareness to the inhale and exhale. As you breathe in, feel the movement of the breath expand your lower ribcage and belly, and as you exhale allow them to contract.

o Continue this for a few rounds.

o Inhale, 2, 3, 4, 5, 6.

o Exhale, 2, 3, 4, 5, 6.

o Notice how you feel in your mind and your body after a couple of minutes.

EVERYDAY STRESS

Often, challenging situations or even mundane events such as being late for a train can literally stop you in your tracks – sending you straight into fight-or-flight mode. Our bodies are designed to maintain balance (the medical term is 'homeostasis'). However, they have not adapted to be triggered constantly and the majority of people are living life in a constant state of low or even high anxiety. Generally, those who are overstressed or anxious breathe more in their upper chests (see pages 14–15). If you are finding it impossible to get any movement in the belly when you breathe, either lie on your belly and make a little pillow with your hands and practise breathing into the floor for a few minutes every day (see pages 251–252) or try Breathing with a sandbag (see opposite).

BREATHING WITH A SANDBAG

By releasing tension with this exercise, you can increase your lung capacity and boost the lymphatic system to move more efficiently, helping detoxify and protect your body from bacteria and other threats to your health. Breathing deeply allows the diaphragm to drop downwards and the ribcage to expand, increasing oxygen flow and helping to slow your heart rate, promoting feelings of calm and relaxation. This is also a great way to activate the diaphragm if you are having difficulty getting the breath lower in your practice.

If you don't have a sandbag to hand, a bag of rice or a heavy book will do.

o Lie down with your knees bent and feet flat on the floor. Allow your arms to rest by your sides.

o Establish a flow of relaxed breathing – feel the breath flowing in and out through your nose.

o Bring your focus to your lower belly. Feel it rise as you inhale and fall as you exhale.

o Let the breath flow with a little pause between the breaths.

o Place the sandbag (or alternative) on your abdomen. Keep your hands on top of the weight so you can feel it moving. You will find that simply placing the weight on the abdomen focuses your attention there. Breathe out and in, raising the weight as you inhale and lowering it

49

as you exhale. Regulate your exhale so that it is relaxed and about the same length as your inhale. This not only strengthens the diaphragm, but tones the muscles of the abdomen as well.

o Let your breath go with a gentle sigh through your nose or mouth and feel your belly coming in. Don't force the air out, simply allow it to flow in and out of your body. Repeat this for a few minutes and notice how you feel.

BREATHING THROUGH THE MENTAL CHATTER

We average 50,000 thoughts a day – the mental chatter never stops. When we go over past events that could have turned out better, or let our anxious internal advisors lead our thoughts about the future, it can make finding the motivation to move forwards and start or complete projects much harder, stalling us from getting anywhere.

While your busy mind ruminates on the past and future, your breath is there in every moment giving you the opportunity to bring your mind and body back to the present. By connecting with your breath you can pull yourself away from the chatter and train your neural pathways to fire and wire together to think more positively. When the pathways between two neurons are repeatedly stimulated, they begin to communicate more effectively. If you're feeding your brain negative thoughts, the pathways for negative thinking become more active and you're much more likely to feel heavier emotions and experience anxiety in your day-to-day life. But, when you take the time to consciously connect with your breath, think about the things you are grateful for and use positive affirmations, the reverse happens and the brain's 'bliss' centre releases dopamine and serotonin, creating feelings of joy and contentment (see more on pages 167–171).

ENERGISING ESPRESSO BREATH

This technique is known as breath of fire or *Kapalabhati* breath and is a great way to boost your energy levels and digestive system, especially if you are feeling sluggish or experiencing that 4 p.m. slump. Before reaching for a coffee or sugar rush to get you through the rest of the afternoon, or to energise you first thing in the morning, try this dynamic abdominal breathing exercise to wake up your mind and get your digestive system moving.

o Sit in an upright position with your spine straight and your hands relaxed on your thighs.

o Take a long, slow inhale through your nose. The exhale is active and the inhale is passive.

o Take a deep breath in.

o As you exhale out through the nose pull your stomach in and pull your navel in towards your spine. Do this as comfortably as you can. Keep one hand on your stomach to feel your abdominal muscles contract.

o As you relax your navel and abdomen, the breath flows automatically. The focus is the exhale as you pull in.

o Take 10–20 such breaths to complete one round. You can increase the rounds with more practice.

o After completing one round, relax with your eyes closed and observe the sensations in your body. Then go for another 2–3 rounds, if you wish.

Note: This exercise creates a very slight CO2 debt in your body but it's not dangerous and helps to move stale air and cleanse the lungs. If you follow it with a slower-breathing pranayama exercise (like alternative nostril breathing, see pages 89–90), your breath will be longer and deeper and it's easier to enter a calm and meditative state.

PEAK PERFORMANCE

Performance is often used to describe a greater sense of productivity, joy and efficiency, so whether you're competing in a sports competition or moving into a new career and feeling nervous about meeting people, presenting your ideas and finding your way, this all falls under the umbrella of performance. So where should you begin if you feel blocked, overwhelmed or hopeless?

Often, we worry too much about what others think of us, constantly looking for approval, wasting our time trying to gauge or change people's opinions. But changing the way you think about yourself is one of the most worthwhile pursuits you can spend time on. By switching your behaviours, your thought patterns and internal chatter, you can alter the way you think and speak to yourself.

Begin with your breath. I encourage you to focus on your breath to become more aware of your thoughts and to avoid descending into a negative spiral of overthinking. Our critical, judgemental minds create internal thoughts such as 'I'm not good enough', 'I don't fit in', 'I can't do this', and leaves us sitting with them. Overthinking can make you lose focus and your sense of who you are, feel fatigued in the day while keeping you awake at night. By letting go of those ruminating thoughts, you create space in the mind for more clarity, joy and positivity.

Try to monitor how much time you spend on screen(s). It can feel overwhelming watching the news, observing social media 'ideals' and reading about climate change.

Far better to ditch the screen for a while and observe the world inside and around you instead. Many of us feel guilty for slowing down, but slowing down is the fastest way to regain balance. On an aircraft they always tell you to put your own oxygen mask on first – you have to look after yourself to be of any use to anyone else. We can make small changes by just taking it one day at a time, remembering to breathe!

BOX BREATHING

Box breathing is a simple relaxation technique that you can do anywhere, including at your desk, in a queue or a coffee shop, to return your breath to its normal rhythm. Its aim is to clear your mind, relax your body and improve focus. When you feel you have no time or space, when you're looking after children, on the school run, facing tight deadlines, cooking or in the shower, this is a perfect go-to rescue remedy. This also helps you switch off from work and relax into the evening.

o Sit with your back supported in a comfortable chair and your feet on the floor.

o Close your eyes. Breathe in through your nose while counting to four slowly. Feel the air enter your lungs.

o Hold your breath while counting slowly to four. Try not to clench your jaw and relax your shoulders. Relax into the breath hold.

o Begin to slowly exhale for four seconds.

o Repeat the inhale, hold and exhale at least three times. Ideally, repeat the three steps for four minutes, or until calm returns. Simply avoid inhaling or exhaling for four seconds.

o If you find the technique challenging, try counting to three instead of four.

ANXIETY &
STRESS

ANXIETY VS STRESS

Anxiety and stress are often confused – they are cousins that look alike but have different root causes. Stress is not always unhealthy – it helps you get the job done and pumps you up ready for a meeting or competition. Anxiety can happen because you feel really passionate about something and the butterflies that you feel are the result of the adrenaline that helps you give your best performance.

Generally, stress is a response to an identifiable external threat that may pass, or that can be dealt with through either fight-or-flight, which is why your internal response primes the body for either or both. Your body is designed to handle stress. However, a build-up of stress over time is not good for you. 'Keep calm and carry on' urges us to bottle up a maelstrom of emotions and continuous low-level stress is now accepted as normal, the result of today's hamster-wheel of inboxes, societal expectations, rolling news and sleep deprivation. The body may be designed to deal with stress, but it needs downtime to process it and if you don't allow yourself that mental space, you will eventually feel it.

Anxiety is more internal – it's what we create for ourselves in response to perceived stress, whether the threat is real or imagined. Immediate threats to our physical safety, job security or health might come and go, but anxiety often sticks around, as we worry about whether the threat might return, remember the difficult past or flash forward to the worst-case scenario.

Anxiety doesn't just come when life is going badly, it can also occur when you are at the height of your career or in a loving relationship. Anxiety can be triggered at different times in your life but rather than trying to push it away, you can listen to your body and gain a deeper understanding of what it is trying to tell you. The symptoms of anxiety can vary from a fluttering tummy, shaky hands, feeling hot and having a tight chest to feeling completely out of control. At its worst it feels like an out-of-body experience you are trying not to let others see, behind a stiff upper lip or a carefully edited Instagram feed.

'Being told to simply "take a deep breath" won't always help unless you also change *how* and *where* you're breathing into.'

Anxiety and stress are natural responses of the autonomic nervous system when processing information that we are under threat. The ancient part of our system that protected us from tigers and wolves can often get triggered and overridden by daily modern life. Although we no longer need our nervous system to protect us from large cats and other sharp-toothed creatures, there are still plenty of 'tigers' in our inboxes and minds. Our stress response doesn't differentiate between a wolf and a seemingly impossible deadline, or even between a 'real' threat versus a perceived one – if our body senses that we're in danger, it triggers red flags throughout our system all the same.

The presence of a frightening stimulus triggers a cascade of hormones which results in adrenaline and cortisol being released. The adrenaline increases heart rate, blood pressure, respiratory rate and diverts blood to the brain – making you more alert – and the skeletal muscles prepare in readiness for fight-or-flight. Adrenaline also causes you to sweat (to manage the heat created by the muscles working hard) and contracts the pupils to sharpen your vision. Cortisol causes glucose to be released from glycogen stores, which is what gives you the 'surge of energy' that is needed for fight-or-flight, but too much of this can create brain fog and fatigue. If we keep hitting that internal alarm system again and again it can lead to chronic stress, panic attacks or chronic anxiety. Lower priority systems such as digestion or reproduction can suffer, generating issues such as irritable bowel syndrome (IBS), constipation, irregular menstrual cycles and low libido.

Anxiety tends to enhance breath-holding or rapid, shallow breaths that come directly from the chest, known as thoracic or chest breathing (see pages 14–17). Many people I work with who have anxiety have tried meditation and breathing exercises but have found that they exacerbate their anxiousness and panic attacks. They find them overwhelming or their breath feels laboured and they feel hungry and gasping for air so they give up. But there's a misunderstanding at play here – being told to simply 'take a deep breath' won't always help unless you also change *how* and *where* you're breathing into.

If you're feeling anxious or panicky and you try to take deeper breaths but the breath is still coming from or limited to your upper torso, with stored tension in your diaphragm, this can make it feel impossible to get a deep diaphragmatic breath in your lower abdominals. This is usually because these muscles have not been used for quite some time, while others have been compensating and overused. The part of our subconscious that associates these feelings with panic will try to control the breath more, disassociate or want to stop. It wants to protect us but we need to gently sweet-talk the feeling using our breath to tell ourselves that we are OK.

How the breath can help

Anxiety is often a memory of a past event that triggers the nervous system or a thought loop catastrophising future events. Sometimes you have to go back through feelings you blocked out in order to process them. The exercises in this chapter are designed to softly move through and

61

uncoil the nervous system without overwhelm and release the overused microscopic muscles which can restrict breathing patterns. There is little point in taking lots of deep breaths if your breath movement is not coming from the belly, so by going slowly and gently and practising daily, you can gradually retrain some of these unhealthy habits you may have picked up along the way.

Using your breath to assure your body you are safe, you can learn to practise holding the feeling of being anxious or stressed until it lessens and becomes lighter and easier to let go. The breath can help alleviate anxiety, but the first steps are to recognise the anxiety, accept it and sit with it. Creating a pause between stimulus and response helps you to remain fully grounded and process stressful events, to recalibrate and reset rather than staying wired. You cannot change all of your circumstances, and there will always be things to worry about, or things you find stressful, but you can change how you respond. Choosing to live in the present is an active process. Rather than burying your feelings or trying to erase a memory, you can learn to fully feel and accept all your experiences and work with them rather than against them.

'The breath can help alleviate anxiety, but the first steps are to recognise the anxiety, accept it and sit with it.'

Creating mental space can help you get to the roots of your anxiety symptoms and help you understand the source of stress first before you attempt to reset. Your mind can't relax if your body feels under threat, but you can teach your brain and nervous system to respond in a healthy way to your environment and triggers, through changing the rhythm, rate and depth of your breath. You can also use breathing exercises on a deeper level as a therapy to recognise the reasons your breath might be dysfunctional, which is usually tied into your nervous system's response to emotions and past events.

No childhood or coming of age is perfectly easy, we all had difficult moments where we felt fear or embarrassment. If you were ever teased for turning scarlet when you had to speak in front of the class, or for forgetting your lines in the nativity play, any time you find yourself in a similar situation as an adult – presenting in front of your colleagues or speaking up at a large meeting – your rational mind knows that you are safe and that things are different but the rest of you hasn't necessarily caught up, and throws you straight back to how you felt in the past, however deeply you've buried the memory. That's why you have to be really gentle. Rather than trying to push the feeling away or getting angry with it, simply allow it and feel it until that little or big memory in your past begins to surrender and your subconscious mind begins to trust that you are safe. Try not to put more pressure on yourself.

BREATHING THROUGH ANXIETY

Anxiety often stops us in our tracks. Your body can sense it before your mind, it tenses up and your breathing pattern changes. By simply acknowledging that these feelings are just energy created by a chemical reaction, you can take hold of them and alter them, rather than allowing them to take hold of you.

Here's a simple exercise to notice the pattern, breathe through it and come out the other side. You can practise this at home or at work and whenever you feel anxiety taking over. This will help to centre you, bringing you back to the present moment.

o Sit up straight and relax your shoulders. Feel your feet connecting to the ground beneath you.

o Become aware of the sensations in your body.

o Pay attention to your surroundings, find two things you can focus on – a chair and a wall, for example. Move your focus back and forth between these two objects for a few seconds while breathing slowly in through your nose and out through your nose.

o Feel the ground or seat beneath you and observe if it is smooth, cold or hot, etc. Now soften your focus or close your eyes.

o Notice the taste in your mouth and the sounds around you. Breathing through your nose, notice if your inhale and exhale feel hot or cold and notice the length of the inhale and exhale.

o Come back to the sensations in your body and bring your attention to your breath. Is your breath moving in your belly? Is it in your chest or perhaps somewhere else?

o Notice your breathing pattern. Is it rapid? Is it shallow? Does it feel restricted? Keep slowing down your breath and bringing the movement of your breath down into your lower body.

o Place your hands on your belly. Take a slow breath in through your nose, allowing a diaphragmatic breath to inflate with enough air to create a slight stretching sensation in your lungs. Slowly exhale.

o Now continue to breathe low into your diaphragm, allowing your belly and ribcage to expand as you inhale, and contract as you exhale. Keep your hands on your lower abdomen and breathe into here. As you inhale your belly expands like a balloon.

o Notice any feelings of anxiety and greet them like old friends, observe the feelings rather than entertaining and feeding them.

o Imagine that your feet are growing roots into the ground. As you breathe in and out, imagine your breath is coming all the way down to your feet.

o Be aware of the sensations in your body as you breathe in and out. Try not to fight the sensations or push them away, just notice and greet them like old friends. Remember these feelings are coming up because your body is trying to protect you.

o Stay with the feelings and let them know that you've got this and you are safe. Stay with them as they will eventually dissipate – don't try to push them away but stay with them in the way you would with a child until they felt safe.

o Breathe through the sensations in your body and as you breathe in and out use these affirmations:

'I let go.'

'I am what I am.'

'I am safe in my body.'

o Continue to breathe deeply into your belly, inhaling and exhaling to stay present with your breath. When you feel ready allow your breath to come back to its normal pattern and notice how you feel.

Tip: This won't necessarily stop anxiety completely after the first practice but by working with the nervous system in this way every time anxiety comes you can retrain your body's reaction and let go of past triggers. Think of each time you practise this exercise as a dress rehearsal. You are seeing the anxiety reaction as a trigger or messenger to work and practise with until you find you can be in the moment without a maelstrom of reactions putting you off and making you forget your lines. In time those triggers will be less activated and easier to control.

MAKING FRIENDS WITH THE TIGERS IN YOUR MIND

What is it that your brain is recording as an external threat, triggering your fight-or-flight response? Your mind is constantly looking for answers to questions – worrying, organising, analysing. If your fight-or-flight response has been activated by a thought, your nervous system isn't aware if this is an actual event or merely a thought, and will immediately trigger your defence mode. The amygdala part of your brain is constantly scanning for danger but by consciously breathing and being aware of how you breathe, you can soothe your nervous system into believing you are safe. You can't control what is happening externally or how others are reacting but you can reframe how it affects you.

There's little doubt that stress can compromise your immune system, so managing stress levels and the high expectations you have of yourself is crucial. By reducing stress, you aid the immune response by reducing inflammation. If inflammation levels are elevated, your lungs, digestive system and all bodily systems are compromised. Flexibility and kindness to yourself is a game changer. Forget FOMO, try saying 'no' more often, be kind to your mind and tune into the messages your body is trying to send you. The more present you are with your breath, the more present you are in your body and the tigers in your mind will begin to seem less agitated and confused. The tigers can be tamed if you treat them gently and rather than being inside you, they can become your allies and walk by your side.

SOLAR PLEXUS ACUPRESSURE

The solar plexus is located just below the ribcage in the upper belly area, above the belly button and below the centre of the ribcage. This space is a collection of two bundles of nerves that intertwine and pass each other at a central location in the abdomen. Its name comes from its resemblance to the sun, with nerves meeting in the centre, creating rays of nerves radiating outwards to many other areas of the body. The solar plexus plays a large role in keeping your organs functioning smoothly, preparing your body to respond to stress (producing a fight-or-flight response) and it is where you experience initial feelings of fear and anger. Some people may feel it pulsating when they feel nervous or excited.

We often find it hard to let go of control and most people I work with have a very tight or even painful solar plexus area. You can help to open your breath and release tension from your diaphragm while stimulating the parasympathetic nervous system by using gentle acupressure here combined with the breath. Practise this whenever you can and notice your breathing pattern becoming freer and more flowing. You can try this using a simple deep diaphragmatic breath.

Practise this exercise now as you are reading.

o Keep your spine straight and body relaxed. Trace down the front midsection of your chest and come under the ribcage – you'll find your solar plexus, which sits just under the diaphragm.

o Bring your right hand to this area and gently use your
   thumb to make circular movements, massaging not on
   the bone but just below the ribcage. Breathe into your
   hand as you massage here – it may feel tight so
   proceed very gently, using your breath to breathe into
   the space and your thumb to help move any tension
   here. Stay with it for a while and try to practise this every
   day or whenever you are stressed or anxious.

BOX BREATHING
FOR CALM AND FOCUS

Box breathing with solar plexus acupressure can help to clear your mind, relax your body and improve focus. If you are feeling nervous before a meeting or presentation this is really great for bringing you back into the moment and clearing your mind of any clutter. For some people, public speaking can bring up fear. You may experience brain freeze, forgetting what you were going to say as your fight-or-flight response shuts down the prefrontal cortex of your brain responsible for communication and memory. This will help to quieten the alarm bells, communicate clearly and make clear decisions.

o Close your eyes. Breathe in through your nose and out through your nose. Focus on your breathing. While working with this technique, practise using the Solar plexus acupressure (see previous exercise) combined with a deep diaphragmatic breath. This will help deepen the practice and make it more effective.

o Relax your shoulders and jaw. Begin to slowly inhale and expand your belly for four seconds.

o Hold your breath for four seconds and relax into the hold.

o Gently let the exhale go and contract your belly for four seconds.

o Hold your breath for four seconds and relax into the hold.

o Repeat steps 2–4 at least six times. Ideally, repeat the
  three steps for four minutes, or until calm returns.

Tip: If you find the technique challenging, try counting to
three instead of four.

DEEP RELEASE BREATH

When you feel fear rising up inside you and are full of nervous energy, you can learn to recognise it as an old pattern and take a moment to listen, get curious and breathe into it. Let fear or anxiety know there is another more powerful force – your breath – and you've got this. This is something you can practise every day or last thing at night. By practising this daily rather than in the moment of stress or anxiety you will find it easier to manage anxiety day to day. Find a quiet space to practise where you won't be interrupted and do this sitting up or lying down. A guided exercise of this is on my podcast *And Breathe*.

The key to this exercise is the pause between breaths and remaining focused and purposeful while waiting until the body inhales. If the mind wanders, bring your focus back to your breath.

o Allow every breath in to be calm and slow. At the top of the inhale, release the air through your open mouth, relax and pause. Patiently wait until the body breathes again.

o Inhale through your nose and then exhale through your mouth. Remember to keep the movement of your breath beginning from the belly. As you inhale, the belly and the ribcage expand and as you exhale, the belly contracts.

o During each pause, allow your body to deeply relax and let go. Allow the pause between each breath to be a time to soften your whole body and release any tension.

o Identify where any tension is in your body, breathe into this area and consciously feel the tightness releasing and letting go.

o Use two fingers to find your breastbone (the bone in the centre of your chest), and then trace down the breastbone until you reach the central point of the ribcage. Guide your finger a couple of centimetres down from the breastbone. Place two fingers on that point and apply gentle pressure on the exhale and then release on the inhale. Make sure your fingers are not on the bone but just below. This is your solar plexus area.

o Repeat affirmations in your head as you breathe in and out: 'I let go', 'I trust and I let go.' Practise this for a minute or two.

o Now let your head fall to the right and hang there and feel the release in the left side of your neck and shoulder. Again apply gentle pressure with two fingers along the trapezius muscle on the top of your shoulder. Use gentle pressure on the exhale and release on the inhale.

o Affirm that: 'I let go of any tension I am holding on to here'. We tend to hold on to responsibility in our shoulders and if we are sat at a desk for a long time, we can feel a build-up of tightness. Give yourself permission to let go of any tension that you may be holding with each exhale.

o Practise this for a minute or two and then repeat on the opposite side. The shoulders should feel freer and lighter as the tension in your neck is released.

o Now bring your head back to the centre and continue inhaling through the nose and letting go of the exhale through the mouth.

o Practise a few more rounds inhaling and then exhaling and waiting for the breath to naturally inhale. On the exhale feel yourself letting go of anything that doesn't serve you.

o Take a deep breath in through your nose and let the exhale go with a big sigh out of your mouth. Do this three more times and notice how your body feels.

THE ART OF LETTING GO

This exercise is simple but effective. It helps to declutter your mind and access parts of the brain that can bring inner peace and bliss. Slow-paced breathing supports the heart and improves stress resilience. When we are focused on a challenging task, when we have too much on our minds, when we are worried about the kids, school, money or ageing parents, we are less flexible and tend to make snap decisions and become more reactive. This exercise can balance and counteract all of that.

This is an exercise you can practise anywhere but ideally in a space where you won't be interrupted. Do it for five minutes or half an hour. The more you practise, the deeper you can go.

o Relax your shoulders and visualise breathing into your heart centre for a while. Breathe slowly and gently in through your nose and out through your nose and move your focus down into your core, just a couple of inches below your belly button. Keep the movement of the breath there.

o Close your eyes, then begin to become aware of your breathing, focusing on the fact that you are breathing. Allow your whole body to relax into the floor beneath you. Visualise your breath coming all the way to your feet. Allow your mind to keep following the breath as you expand your focus inwards, letting go of the outside world.

- Notice any feelings, sounds and sensations as you continue to focus on the inhale and exhale.

- Leave all your thoughts behind and use the affirmation 'I let go' with each inhale and exhale.

- Imagine your breath arising from within you: breathe into your right side, your left side, above and below you. Imagine your breath moving beyond your skin, out into the universe and keep repeating the mantra 'I let go'.

- As you breathe in and out, draw the movement all the way down to your hips and pelvis, where you have little diaphragm-like muscles in the pelvis correlating with your main diaphragm.

- Stay with your breath and repeat the affirmation 'I let go': on the inhale 'I let' and on the exhale 'go'.

- Keep your focus here and allow yourself to travel with the breath and the affirmation. This can take you deeper and deeper, away from your mind and help to expand your inner awareness.

- When you feel ready, begin to bring your breathing back to its normal pattern. Become aware of your surroundings and open your eyes. Notice how you feel.

MENTAL &
EMOTIONAL
RESILIENCE

ACCEPTANCE AND LETTING GO

Mental and emotional resilience comes through
acceptance. While you're not always able to control life's
ups and downs, by embracing emotional experiences, you
will be stronger in your foundations. Less dependent on
ticking off successes, being loved by others or receiving
nods of approval in order to feel good. Breathing exercises
remind you to unlearn what you think you know and
un-become who you think you are. Allow yourself to
unravel and get comfortable with being uncomfortable.
Know it's OK to not always feel OK, to change direction
and let go of parts of your life that no longer serve you.

Travelling inwards can at times make you hold your breath
and resist feeling. The subconscious mind wants to protect
you and tell you that you'd be safer if you just turned back,
so you stay in the loop of a story that limits possibilities. If
you're feeling overwhelmed by obstacles, it's harder to
move forwards but by keeping your breath flowing you
can move more easily through 'freeze' mode.

The nature of breathwork is not to force an outcome but
to encourage you to connect to your inner compass and

make space to let new energy in. Knowing yourself deeply through each heartbeat and breath can help you to accept when something in your life no longer serves a purpose and find the courage and grace to release it. Maybe you want to let go of old habits, relationships, a career or a lifestyle. More often than not, you might struggle to take the first step, to start that new diet, stop feeling anxious or practise a daily fitness routine – and it's not because you just forgot. There's a subconscious process that controls every action and decision you take. Understanding your behaviours, patterns and fears is the first step to making change. All behavioural patterns have triggers which come in many shapes and sizes: environmental, social, mental and emotional. This is where it can get challenging. It's one thing to say you want something but the work to get there can feel rocky and unfamiliar, especially when your ego is shouting at you not to give up the familiar. You can question your decisions if you feel a sense of loss, even if the change is in your best interests in the long term. When you work in harmony with your breath you bring in more balance and slowly, with patience and time breathwork becomes part of daily life. Whatever you are doing or not doing, you have an opportunity in every moment to come back into balance by using your breath.

'Knowing yourself deeply
through each breath
can help you to accept
when something in your life
no longer serves a purpose
and find the courage and
grace to release it.

In the indigenous language Quechua, spoken primarily in the Peruvian Andes, the word 'ayni' means 'all things in the right balance', whether it's in the environment or your body. The concept of *ayni* includes reciprocity with nature because nature is part of us; it's the source of life and of everything that keeps us alive and nurtures us, and it is therefore our duty to reciprocate. This way of thinking means that you recognise when something is out of balance in the world around you and know you must balance something within you. Balance yourself within, then witness the shift around you; your thoughts and actions and your body's response.

By embodying this approach, you can regulate and monitor your wellbeing by recognising the signs and symptoms of burnout and taking steps to reduce its harmful effects. Sometimes we need to be reminded that we are human beings, not human doings, and by connecting to our breath we remember how we are able to adapt and respond to different environments and circumstances.

BRING BACK BALANCE BREATH

If your emotions are spiralling or you have too many tabs open in your brain and need to declutter your mind, this exercise is great to bring back balance and give yourself the space to breathe.

o Feel the ground beneath your feet and become aware of your breath. As you inhale, expand and breathe deeply into your belly. As you exhale, feel your feet rooting into the ground.

o Notice your breath and any sensations in your body. Keep focusing on these sensations. Allow your mind to follow the movement of the inhale and exhale.

o Breathe into your toes and visualise them making roots into the ground. Take a few deep breaths.

o Breathe in for a count of four and out for a count of eight. Breathing in through your nose and out through pursed lips.

o Close your eyes and connect your breath to your heartbeat. Bring your awareness into your heart space.

o Allow all your awareness to drift into your body. Feel the temperature of the sun on your skin. Listen to the sounds around you. Inhale and stretch your arms up to the sky, then bring them down slowly with the exhale. Repeat, continuing to breathe in for four as you raise

81

your arms up and breathe out for eight as your arms
come down.

o Breathe fully, deeply and slowly and keep letting go of
your thoughts.

The vagus nerve

The vagus nerve is one of the most important parts of the parasympathetic nervous system (see page 27) and the most complex of all our nerves. In Latin 'vagus' means 'wanderer' and this nerve is so called because it wanders throughout the body connecting the brain to the tongue, pharynx, vocal cords, lungs, heart, stomach, nervous system and intestines as well as glands that produce enzymes and hormones influencing digestion and metabolism.

As such it is vital to the mind-body connection. The key to mental and emotional resilience is developing strong vagal tone which can activate the parasympathetic pathways of your nervous system on command. Vagal tone becomes weak when you have unresolved trauma in the body and low vagal tone is linked to chronic inflammation, high blood pressure, anxiety, depression, lack of focus, chronic illness and digestive issues. It also keeps you stuck in fight-or-flight mode where your body believes you are in a state of constant threat. Your breath is a tool that you can use to turn down the stress response in your body and develop a healthy vagal tone that can help you switch between the parasympathetic nervous system, which regulates your digestion, reproduction and endocrine systems while slowing down the heart rate, and the sympathetic nervous system when required.

CALMING BREATH

This breathing exercise will, with regular practice, help you feel calmer and more focused and can also be good for pain relief. When you're experiencing stress, anxiety, depression or conflict, breathing consciously will help you to bounce back.

It can be practised sitting up in a comfortable chair or in bed, propped up at a 45-degree angle with pillows. It's an effective way to fall back to sleep if you wake in the night and can also be practised lying down.

o Make sure you are in a warm room or covered with a blanket. Maximum comfort is required so indulge yourself.

o Close your eyes, relax your body and tune in to your breath. Notice how it is moving and bring the movement into your belly. The belly expands on the inhale and contracts on the exhale.

o Start using an ocean or 'ujjayi' breath by drawing your breath to the back of your sinus cavity so you can feel it in the top and back of your throat.

o Exhale through your mouth with a soft 'Haaa' sound, like you are misting a mirror. Allow your exhale to last longer than your inhale and try not to force or push either.

o On the tenth inhale, pause the inhalation for four seconds. Relax into the hold.

o Exhale slowly through your mouth, then hold the exhale for 3–4 seconds.

o Repeat the inhale and exhale for another round of ten without any holding, using the ocean breath and letting go with a 'Haaa' sound on your exhale.

o Return to your natural breathing rhythm and allow your vagal system to reset. Notice any changes and when you are ready, soften your focus and open your eyes.

MARK'S STORY

Mark Whittle is a life coach, has a no.1 podcast *Take Flight* and a genuine passion for helping others become the best version of themselves. He came to see me after living with chronic fatigue syndrome (CFS), which he has overcome using breathing exercises alongside other techniques.

I was always *on*. I was always *doing*. I was always chasing the next *win* or dopamine *high*. Until I couldn't.

In 2013, I boarded a plane at John Glenn Columbus International Airport as I'd spent the previous two years living and playing professional football or 'soccer' in Ohio. For those two years I kept up a gruelling schedule, training every day, sometimes twice, and playing competitively whenever the fixtures dictated. Often three matches a week. At the same time I kept up an even more demanding social schedule. Four heavy nights out a week was not uncommon. I was young, excitable, living my dream and not considering the implications this would have on my future.

Six weeks after landing in London I started to feel really unwell. My joints ached, at times I had a fever, I would wake up with my head pounding and I had never felt so tired. 'It must be the flu,' I thought. I wasn't used to being ill, so I treated my recovery like I would a typical hangover – drinking lots of water and watching films on the sofa. This approach worked for the first day or two, but five years on I was still suffering from what would eventually be diagnosed as chronic fatigue syndrome (CFS). Here started my journey back to health and self.

I was finally, loosely, diagnosed with CFS two years into having symptoms. I would go through awful spells feeling like I couldn't leave my flat for six weeks, followed soon after by feeling fairly healthy for close to a month. One month I even ran the London marathon! But with the symptoms so consistent I grudgingly decided to retire from my one true love, football, and then began uncharacteristically declining most social invites. At this point, I also chose to use all of my good days to read, research and experiment with any ways I could to start to feel healthier. Early on in my journey my brother introduced me to Transcendental Meditation. It was my first experience of any spiritual practice and I loved it. This was an important step in my journey as I got used to the idea of spending time with myself. Meditation allowed me to quieten some of my internal dialogue and to start to take back control of my thoughts.

The most pivotal moment, however, was two years after I'd started practising meditation. One of my best friends had recently been to a holotropic breathwork session; he had visions, he cried and 'came out the room a different person'. I was sceptical, but prepared to try anything. My worry about my symptoms had turned into anxiety and I was experiencing quite low mental health for the first time in my life. I'd read that breathwork could help alleviate stress and anxiety, so I was keen to try it. We immediately booked on to a session that Rebecca was running later that month.

I arrived excited yet curious, but in hindsight I was in no way prepared for what was about to happen. I hadn't cried in years, but within ten minutes I was sobbing on the floor. I would later find out this was energy or emotion which had been stored in my body and was finally being released. It felt like I'd lifted a bottle cap and everything I'd been holding on to came out. The biggest lesson was how these tears were uncontrollable, and that if I wanted to feel at peace I had to let go. Let go of expectation. Let go of perfection. Let go of stored negative emotion.

I continued to practise breathwork with Rebecca both in group settings and later one-to-one. The more I practised, the more I found that breathing also removed fear and allowed me to get to the heart of what I was chasing. Or more accurately, what I was running away from. I was able to consider and address things that I had never been prepared to before, and that took such a weight off my shoulders. I even felt the fear dissipate around ideas I'd been holding on to and not yet acted on. For example, starting a podcast, which has now become my full-time job. Three years into my breathwork journey and my fatigue is almost gone. I still suffer from time to time, but I now recognise the signs. I can train in the gym again, box and am working towards having the impact I want to have in the world.

'Breathing well stimulates the body to work better, to move the lymphatic system freely and detox.'

ALTERNATIVE NOSTRIL BREATHING

Also known as *Nadi Shodhana* in Sanskrit, which roughly translates to 'clearing the channels of circulation'. Estimates suggest that the philosophy behind this practice dates back to 700 BC. This is a simple and powerful technique often practiced as part of yoga. Whenever you are finding it hard to focus or make important decisions, alternative nostril breathing helps you to feel grounded and more resilient. The right and left nostrils have their own control centres, which communicate with the cardiovascular system and signal the brain to produce chemicals that alter mood and emotions. When breathing through the right nostril, you stimulate the sympathetic nervous system SNS (see page 27), which puts you in an elevated state of vigilance and alert. This feeds more blood to the left side of the brain's prefrontal cortex area, associated with practical decision-making and logistical and analytical thinking. Inhaling through the left nostril stimulates your parasympatheic nervous system PNS (see page 27), which promotes a more relaxed, digestive state and lowers body temperature. The blood flow shifts to the right side of the prefrontal cortex, which stimulates creative thinking, imagination and intuition.

o This is best performed sitting, so get comfortable, keeping your spine straight. Visualise a string coming out of the centre of your head, drawing it up towards the sky. Remember to use a diaphragmatic breath (see pages 29–30).

o Try to match the length of your inhales, pauses and exhales and don't force your breath. Start to inhale for a count of three, hold for three, exhale for three, hold for three. Slowly increase the count as you refine your practice.

o Place your left hand, palm up, on your lap and your right hand just in front of your nose.

o Bring your right index and middle fingers to rest lightly between your eyebrows. The fingers you'll be actively using are the thumb and ring finger.

o Close your eyes and take a deep breath in and out through your nose.

o Close your right nostril with your right thumb. Inhale slowly and steadily through your left nostril.

o Close your left nostril with your ring finger so both nostrils are held closed; hold your breath at the top of the inhale with a little pause.

o Open your right nostril and release your breath gently through your right nostril; pause again at the end of the exhale.

o Inhale through your right nostril slowly and gently. Hold both nostrils closed (with ring finger and thumb).

o Open your left nostril and exhale slowly through your left nostril. Pause briefly. Inhale slowly and steadily through your left nostril. Close your left nostril with your ring finger so both nostrils are held closed; hold your breath at the top of the inhale and pause.

o Continue for a couple of minutes and practise whenever you feel the need for balance.

BE MORE TORTOISE

Being in constant survival mode to power through life without taking time out to recalibrate and recharge is common. Proving your worth, importance and busy-ness to yourself and others is a modern human trait. How many conversations have you had with family, colleagues and friends about what a busy day is ahead? Although we have not evolved to go at the speed of machines, you may catch yourself regularly putting pressure on yourself to do so. Rather than speed-walking through life, how about getting busy practising stillness? Every day let kindness be the starting block. Kindness to yourself, your thoughts and to others.

A tortoise breathes four times a minute and can live to be well over a hundred years old. If we take away the obvious differences in the respiratory needs of humans and tortoises and simply look at the message, slowing down your respiratory rate can add higher quality to your life. If you slow down your breath, you naturally take a deeper breath. When you slow down, you are able to let go of dizzying thoughts and create space to really listen to your body. Stillness is how to stay sane when all around feels out of control. Attention is the opposite of distraction. Slowing down your breath brings stillness and attention and in this quietness you can intuitively recognise what is best for you to restore and reset.

HEAD AND NECK TENSION RELEASE

This restorative self-massage breath exercise is relaxing and effective. It can be practised any time, but is particularly good after a long day when you're in need of a wind-down and some self-care. If you find yourself spending a lot of time on a screen at your desk, this helps to relieve any tension accumulated from a sedentary day of concentrating while slouching forwards. You can also practise this in bed if you have been feeling fatigued or unwell.

o Find a peaceful space and take a few moments to centre yourself. Focus on your breath and feel your feet on the ground.

o Open your mouth, stretch your jaw and move your lips. Pull as many faces as possible in all directions. Focus on the breath being slow and mindful.

o Tap your face briskly with your fingertips. This improves blood supply to the skin and exercises the facial muscles.

o Drum gently all over your scalp with loose fists.

o Use your fingers and thumbs to trace and massage your jawline.

o Use your fingers and thumbs to gently pinch up and around your ears. Massage around your ears and earlobes.

o Place your hands on the back of your neck and massage up and down, keeping your breath flowing.

○ Spread the fingers of both hands on your scalp with your thumbs tucked under the base of the skull. Here you will find the occipital muscles. Massage deeply into this whole area. Connect to your breath as you do this and breathe slowly and deeply. Feel the release.

FORGIVING THE PAST

You can't change the past but you can stop carrying it around with you. This doesn't mean accepting or excusing behaviour but letting it go and preventing it from accumulating into resentment and bitterness.

Setting boundaries means defining what you can or cannot accept. You have to authentically feel you can forgive and decide when you are ready to do so, there is no time limit. Breathwork is the most powerful route I have witnessed to achieving forgiveness and letting go of blame while still embracing vulnerability and strength. When you free yourself from the stories of the past you can be here right now where everything is as it should be. Start with your breath.

BREATHE AND FORGIVE

Forgiveness isn't a switch. Forgiveness is a process to be respected, observed and not rushed. With this exercise adapted from the teachings of Thich Nhat Hanh, you can ground yourself to better navigate through emotional triggers and thoughts from your past.

o Find a peaceful space to practise. Stand up straight, with your feet hip distance apart and swing your arms, moving your torso gently from right to left while feeling and thinking about the situation that requires forgiveness.

o Observe the emotions and thoughts that accompany the past hurt while focusing on the movement. Keep the breath rhythmic and flowing.

o Come back to stillness. Sit down in a comfortable chair or on the floor. Breathe in as deeply as you can and let go of the exhale as far as you can.

o When you are ready, start to notice any sensations in your body.

o Bring your attention to your thoughts. Watching the thoughts and allowing them to pass.

o When you are ready, bring your attention to any emotions that arise. Letting go, letting be. Allowing whatever is present to be just as it is.

o Bring to mind a situation that feels unresolved. See who is there in your mind and stay with your breath. Trust yourself to feel forgiveness when it feels right for you, without getting lost in the story of what may have happened. Try not to put any expectation on yourself to feel forgiveness then and there. Just be with your feelings and stay with your breath, sending love and compassion into your heart. Saying:

'I give myself permission to forgive and let go.'

'I release myself and others from the story.'

'I can feel my breath and my breathing feels free.'

o Take a few moments to transition, to let go of any images or thoughts. Notice how you feel. Focus on your body and your breath. Take a few deep breaths. Practise this as often as you like and perhaps write down how you feel afterwards or take some time to be with your thoughts on a walk or with a cup of tea.

TRAUMA

TRAUMA

Most of us have experienced mental, emotional or physical trauma on some level, which can restrict our breathing and capacity to feel. We may distract, numb, check out or disassociate when experiencing trauma or when triggered by past trauma. This chapter is a gentle entry into understanding how you can release both the big and little traumas held in your body. I always recommend going slowly and working at your own pace. Resilience comes from understanding and building awareness when letting your guard down and accepting the parts of yourself that may feel vulnerable or want to disassociate, understanding them and taking care of them. The breath is your anchor to bring awareness to your senses, which at times can feel overwhelming.

What story is hiding underneath the tension? Suppressed emotion and trauma gets stored in the cells, tissues, jaw, hips and shoulders. When trauma isn't processed, it can start to control your daily life. Cutting people off, shutting parts of yourself down. In situations where you are safe, the body can still go into panic or shut down mode because of past memories the body hasn't computed due to unprocessed trauma.

Animals instinctively shake to discharge the effects of being chased by predators and we are wired in the same way as our four-legged friends. This cycle is called the fight, flight or freeze response. And every time you experience danger, this cycle gets triggered. It's a fantastic tool to ensure our survival. There is one problem, however. Many of us are experiencing fight, flight or freeze on a daily basis and don't process this afterwards. The danger might not be a tiger, but the traffic jam making you late for work, the impending economic crisis, disruption in the home, etc. These 'dangers' can all trigger your nervous system into survival mode. They are also much more abstract and therefore less tangible, which means that often you don't even notice you are in a state of fight-or-flight because society normalises it. And it therefore invalidates the need for discharge or emotional release. Trauma results from the 'freeze' energy in your body, energy that hasn't had the chance to complete its cycle and from how effectively your nervous system is able to deal with this.

Breathing through old triggers

'What' happened to you doesn't necessarily need to define you and you don't have to carry it with you all your life. Giving yourself space and time to feel your feelings is one of the healthiest and most productive things you can do. Connecting with your breath is the way back home to your senses and intuition. It is the starting block to healing. Healing the past, healing trauma, healing wounds, betrayal, abuse, judgement, abandonment and letting go of any armour that is trying to protect you but also holding you back. When you free your body from trauma, you are able to listen more easily to your intuition and trust your gut. When you do the 'work', your relationship with yourself improves and your relationships with others can shift. Self-care isn't selfish; putting yourself first means that you are committing to do the work and aren't carrying around the residue of hurt and wounding from buried trauma, accidentally and unconsciously inflicting this on others. You also give yourself permission to be open to higher vibrational feelings such as joy and love.

Fear is a very old pattern and often it stops us in our tracks. You can feel your body reacting and your breathing pattern changing but by remembering that it is simply energy, you can take hold of it and alter the feeling rather than allowing it to take hold of you. Here's a simple exercise to notice the pattern, breathe through it and come out the other side.

REFRAMING THE STORY

Use this exercise to bring you into the present moment and notice any feelings that are arising. You may have had a confrontation with someone or read an email that made you feel nervous about a social or work situation. Is it the email that is triggering you, or a past event that you haven't processed? Track your feelings and be aware of the sensations in your body as you take time to breathe into them. Most importantly, be gentle and cradle these feelings like you would a child who didn't feel safe or understood.

This exercise can be practised sitting up or lying down.

o Become aware of the feelings and sensations in your body. Track them and get curious: are they in your belly, in your chest or somewhere else? Notice your breathing pattern – is it rapid? Is it shallow? Does it feel restricted?

o Now, breathe low into the lungs using your diaphragm, allowing your belly and ribcage to expand as you inhale and contract as you exhale.

o Notice any feelings and greet them like old friends, become the observer rather than entertaining or analysing these feelings.

o Feel your feet on the ground and imagine that they are growing roots deep into the ground giving you a strong foundation.

o As you breathe in and out, visualise the breath coming all the way down to your feet. Be aware of

the sensations in your body as you breathe in and
breathe out.

o Try not to fight or resist the sensations or push them
away – just notice them. Breathe through and into the
sensations in your body as you inhale and exhale. Like a
tree you are rooted.

o Breathe in and let your body know 'I am safe in my
body'. Use affirmations, such as 'It's safe to feel all my
feelings'.

o Continue to breathe deeply into your belly, inhaling and
exhaling, and stay present with your breath. Continue
this practice for as long as it feels comfortable.

WHOLE BODY MUSCLE
TENSING AND RELAXING

This exercise stimulates the parasympathetic nervous system (see page 27) while engaging the muscles of the entire body. This can help you when you can't shift pent-up tension or you're feeling frozen from a challenging situation. If you're facing anything that is anxiety provoking, like a meeting or social engagement, this exercise can be done quickly beforehand.

This exercise can be done lying down or sitting up, but it's more effective lying down.

o Take a deep breath in through your mouth; visualise filling up your lungs.

o Hold your breath. Then close your mouth and take in another sip on the inhale and then another.

o While holding your breath, engage your perineum (the space between the genitals and anus) and your core and throat area, and keep the breath held.

o Tense or scrunch up your face, nose, eyes, hands, feet, stomach, buttocks, thighs and legs. Count 5–10 seconds while holding your breath and keeping all muscles tense.

o Relax everything, let go of all the tension in your muscles and slowly let your exhale go. Repeat 3–4 times.

Past trauma

When people think of trauma they tend to think of dramatic situations like abuse or living in a war zone, but smaller incidents such as dealing with ill health, break-ups, or even losing a job or leaving a community that's important to you can also have a deep impact. If authority let you down as a child or you felt unloved, abandoned, rejected or ignored, you can carry these experiences into later life. Something like being scared by a big dog, getting lost in a crowd or being laughed at in school may not seem like a life-altering event in childhood, but it can lead to feeling a lack of your basic primal needs, such as reassurance, attention, love, security and trust, being met.

If as a child you did not experience feeling valued for who you were, you may desperately seek to prove your value through what and how much you do. If your early environment was unpredictable or hurtful, you may develop a pattern in your body and how you perceive the world in which you perceive threat even when there isn't any. Your internal world's relationship with the external world can become tilted.

If you haven't processed trauma, the event can be stored in your body as trauma memory which can be tapped back into when retriggered. So, if your house was broken into when you were little, for example, when you are older you might be triggered when there are sounds outside at night that set off hyperarousal because your brain and body have not processed that trauma and are still on high alert.

By sitting with the emotions, you can breathe into and through uncomfortable feelings. We can be masters of distracting, numbing out and keeping ourselves busy to avoid our feelings. By sitting with your feelings in the way you would sit with a child who was upset or scared, you are able to build trust and a better relationship with yourself.

FINDING A SAFE SPACE

This self-soothing exercise helps you to lean into your senses and be in the present moment. To experience the difference between 'thinking mode' versus 'feeling mode' and strengthen your ability to discern deeper levels of feeling.

Somatic therapy often utilises touch because it more directly intervenes with the nervous system. Touch can include self-touch to provide a sense of being safe here in the room. Take your time with each of the steps as when you experience emotional arousal from being triggered it can be difficult to contain the energy of those emotions. This exercise keeps you grounded by re-establishing a sense of feeling safe in your body. You can practise this sitting or lying down.

o Take a moment to feel the ground beneath you, the temperature of the room and notice your surroundings and sounds.

o Focus on any feelings in your body. Is there any heaviness or lightness or tightness?

o Place your right hand below your left armpit, holding the side of your chest. Breathe into your hand, slowly and mindfully.

o Place your left hand on your right shoulder and breathe into your hand, keeping your focus here for a while.

o Notice the feelings under your right and left hands. Does your body feel warm? Do your shoulders feel tense or relaxed? Is your skin or clothing smooth or cold? Can you feel your pulse or heartbeat? Do you experience a sense of comfort or support from your hands? Close your eyes and notice how the rest of your body responds to this.

o Scan your body and find a space in your body that feels safe and even more held. It may be your stomach or lower back or shoulders. Stay with that space, and keep breathing gently into that space, inhaling through your nose and exhaling through your mouth. You can come back to this space whenever you need to feel grounded.

o Take your time with each of these steps, so that you spend at least a minute on the entire exercise. Keep your breathing slow and mindful.

o Take a moment and notice your overall experience. Move your feet on the floor, moving and shifting until you feel really connected to the floor.

o Once you have practised this exercise a few times and are familiar with it, you can skip straight to closing your eyes and go to your safe space. Play with the exercise and use your intuition to see how it works best for you.

REBECCA'S STORY

When Rebecca first came to see me, the whole right side of her body was in pain. Her breath pattern was frozen and with little movement of the breath in her body. Rebecca has been in survival mode for most of her life. When I was working with her at first, combining bodywork and breathing exercises it was important, as with all clients, to develop a deep trust. Her mind trusted me but her body was in defence mode. By working slowly and gently with movement and gentle acupressure, over time her body felt safe enough to be supported and let go. Rebecca works supporting and empowering women in business. She is one of the most courageous and kind people I know.

My story is not unusual. It's not a tale of the greatest suffering but it's one that, until recently, has affected my experience of life and the choices I have made. I was not conceived from, or born into, love or family. I was born to two people, trapped by circumstance, who didn't want each other or a child. They each operated from the extreme ends of hot and cold. My father was permanently shut down, absent and sulking. My mother was volatile and full of rage, drowning in grief and mental ill-health. When I was a small baby, the police were called to our house when my mother was found dangling me out of a top floor window, threatening to drop me if I didn't stop crying. So started my early years.

I imagine it was from this point that I became an exceptionally good baby and child. By 'good' this meant quiet, not drawing attention, not asking for anything, trying

to pre-empt drama and not breathing too loudly
(I remember clearly the regular slaps across the face
when my breathing irritated my mother). Physical affection
was rare and something to be scared of. Throughout my
life, my mum wore her lack of fondness and interest in
children like a badge: 'I don't like children, and I didn't
want this one'. My parent's unhappiness played out for
four years, and not one picture or memory exists of us as
family from this time. There are a handful of pictures of me,
always on my own, always looking serious. My parents
spent the first few years of my life making plans to escape.
For my mother, this involved having a very public affair
with a married man. My father went to sea, remarried and
was rarely seen again. This was just the beginning.

In spring 2019, I was silently making contact with rock
bottom. I've been praised throughout my life for an ability
to remain swan-like when faced with challenges, and this
time was no different. On the surface, I was my usual
in-control self, but underneath I was flooded with darkness.
Overwhelmed with stress and past trauma, I defaulted to a
numbed-out state in order to function. An addiction to
work had become a way of checking out. An acceptable
replacement for earlier, more hedonistic, means. Haunted
by a fear of unravelling, I berated myself constantly. I told
myself that if I could just do more, be more, achieve more,
then maybe I might finally outrun myself. It was exhausting.

It was living in this state of constant stress, running a
company while also being the principle carer for my
daughters, that I knew something had to give. I started

talking therapy, and though it was beneficial on many levels, I found the sessions physically debilitating. Revisiting past trauma triggered powerful waves of fear, shame and anxiety. We would head into the story and then I would panic and detach. I left the sessions in intense discomfort and often hyperventilated afterwards. I understood why this cycle was happening, but I didn't have the tools to tackle it. And so to be able to continue with the sessions, I did what I had always done; rationalised, disassociated and shut down.

It was at this point that I came across breathwork. A podcast on a crowded commute introduced me to the therapeutic benefits of learning how to breathe. As I listened to Rebecca talk about breathwork, I could see how it might help me. I knew I had rogue breathing patterns. I believe I've held my breath since early childhood, and I knew enough to know that these patterns were connected in some way to my anxiety symptoms.

Not knowing what to expect, I put my trust in Rebecca. I lay down and followed her voice. That first session of connected breathing was unlike anything I had ever experienced. It was physically challenging and the perfectionist in me worried that I wouldn't be able to do it correctly. Soon, though, as the breath moved, I was experiencing tingling in my limbs, energy moving around my body, temperature changes and what felt like a heightened state of awareness. Yet it was the emotional unfolding which I'll never forget. In an entirely lucid state, I experienced forgotten memories and intense feelings of grief, shock and sadness.

With the physical process of maintaining the connected breathing keeping me present, I had no choice but to let the emotions in, trusting Rebecca to guide me through the process and out the other side. Afterwards, I felt a flutter of inner peace for the first time. And so started my journey with breathwork.

I have started to heal some very raw and hidden areas of my life. I have been able to slowly unpack and process the emotional and physical residues of childhood trauma, rape and depression in a way that feels kind and manageable to my mind and body. The magic of this work is that it never feels more than I can handle in the moment and I am learning to feel safe in myself. Having the foundations of a regular breathing practice helps me create the impetus and space I need to get out of my head and out of the past when it all gets too much, and to let go of the things that no longer serve me. I can find the present more easily and in doing so more freely trust that storms will pass in time.

Life is far from perfect, and challenges still persist. There is still much for me to learn, much for me to let go of. But the benefits of breathwork have already had a profound impact on my life. I leave each breathing session with greater clarity, a desire to forgive (both others and myself) and a true desire to stop holding so tightly. The moments of stillness and reflection created in this practice have supported a period of personal and spiritual growth that may not have had happened otherwise.

We should all be grateful to our breath for keeping us alive. The space breathwork creates is helping me accept who I am. I can finally feel the need to outrun me, or find a different version of me, slowly ebbing away. This is a beautiful gift and for this I am truly grateful.

WORKING THROUGH TRAUMA WITH A BREATH THERAPIST

When working with clients and trauma it is important for any therapist to understand that breathing exercises can bring up past experiences and, if not held well, can retraumatise. You can't simply read a book about trauma and then teach how to heal it – it takes years of practice and experience. Over my years of working with the breath, I have seen people fast-track training and using methods that can activate trauma immediately and this can be very dangerous. If you are working with a breathworker or coach and it doesn't feel comfortable, always go with your gut and remember it is your body and your right to stop the session whenever you choose. If there is overwhelming trauma coming up, it is advisable to work with a certified therapist who can create a safe space to help you navigate through it.

SHAKE IT OUT

Shaking is a natural response to extreme stress. It can be a good form of therapy as rather than pushing feelings down, you can shake them off. When you have held tension and trauma, parts of the brain become stuck in defensive strategies, making you tight and contracted – prepared for fight-or-flight or freezing the body. Shaking while working with your breath is a safe and easy way of releasing tension and waking up your body.

o Begin standing, allowing your focus to soften and take some deep breaths in and out through your nose.

o Rise up slowly on to your toes, and then drop back down to your heels. Repeat this slowly and methodically.

o Bring your attention to the effect it has on your hips and lower back. Try to let them relax. Do this a few times.

o Come back to standing and take five more deep breaths.

o Slightly bending the knees, gently bounce. Create a soft shaking and bouncing motion in your knees and legs. Imagine this shaking can gently rock through your whole body, through your hips, up to your shoulders, and even your neck.

o Try to relax your jaw, lower back and tailbone, as if the base of your spine is really heavy. Do this for a minute or so.

o Stand still again, and let your hands come to rest on the front of your thighs. You might notice little tremors or shudders in your body, which might feel unusual at first, but allow them to travel through you as your body releases tension.

o Now come down on to the floor and lie on your back with the soles of feet together, knees bent out to the sides. Take some breaths here and become aware of the ground supporting you. Close your eyes.

o Every couple of minutes bring your knees towards each other inch by inch and hold. As the inner thigh muscles engage at some point, you will notice a slight tremble. Simply stay with the trembling sensation and allow it to happen.

o Bring your knees closer and notice if the shaking becomes stronger. Don't hold your breath and simply be with the shaking. You may notice other parts of your body begin to shake.

o When you feel ready, allow your legs to come down, stay with your breath for a while and notice how you feel.

GRIEF

Speaking about grief can be a real conversation stopper. It can make people feel awkward and uncomfortable. Sometimes people aren't ready or willing to share their rage, anger, sadness, guilt and all the feelings that come with grief, and are often encouraged to move on rather than to sit with it and feel it.

Grieving is not something in many cultures we are shown or guided to express. Grief comes in many forms, it's not just about losing someone but it can also be a feeling of losing a part of ourselves, a way of life, the end of a relationship, loss of direction, paths we didn't walk, a career or what we thought our future would look like. It makes us want to shut down and protect our hearts and hold our breath, yet the breath is the necessary current we need to carry us through.

QIGONG GENTLE SWAY

Qigong is a concept from traditional Chinese culture that is roughly translated as "vital energy cultivation". It is considered and practiced as a beautiful art by countless people all over the world. In Chinese medicine, grief is the emotion carried by the lungs. Many of us have self-doubt around fully expressing heavier emotions as we don't want to be a burden on others or look like we cannot cope. When suppressing feelings it can feel weighty. When grief is unprocessed, depression and an inability to let go can arise. Since our lungs control the flow of energy in our bodies, it's important that we give ourselves time to grieve and breathe through painful events rather than bottling them up. This exercise helps to keep present with the movement and the feeling. Twisting from the waist also massages your internal organs and releases tension in the tummy.

o Feel your feet on the ground and soften your focus.

o Bring the breath low and breathe softly through your nose.

o Begin to gently bounce by bending your knees.

o Keep your knees slightly bent and come back to stillness.

o Move your arms in a gentle swinging motion for a few minutes. The motion itself is initiated from your waist. Allow your head to follow the movement of your arms. Close your eyes.

- As you twist to the left inhale and exhale as you twist to the right.

- Twist from your waist. Inhale and exhale to the rhythm of the swinging motion.

- Just being with the motion and movement and feeling the ground beneath you.

- Notice how you feel after a few minutes. You may experience a slight shift in energy or mood.

Time to grieve

Whenever you feel heavy emotions such as grief or anger, allow your inner parent to be the lighthouse to guide the emotions of your inner child. Let them know that they are safe and they are loved and you are listening to whatever it is that needs to be held and heard. Create a space in between the inhale and exhale to be present with these feelings. Stay with your breath and it will guide you through. We don't need to suppress everything we feel. We don't have to be positive all the time. It's not bad to feel sad or angry. To feel is to be human.

Massage, touch, breathing exercises or self-massage are all supportive ways to feel held. Many experiences in life that bring grief can feel like being trapped or stuck. Using your body to express your grief by walking in nature or running, dancing or doing some gentle yoga can take you beyond words by simply being present and moving with the feeling. Be kind to your heart and take your time.

DEEPENING YOUR SENSES

Take a moment to sit back and feel all of your emotions. When you acknowledge loss, failures and disappointments, you free yourself from attachments and stories you feel you have to carry. This doesn't mean you have to forget or even forgive if you don't feel ready yet, it simply creates space to allow you to breathe into all aspects of your life until your path becomes clearer.

o Close your eyes or focus on a spot on the floor, then begin to become aware of your breathing, focusing on the fact that you are breathing.

o Notice your breath moving in and out, specifically as it enters and leaves the tips of your nostrils.

o Follow your breath from this point of focus, in and out, for a minimum of ten cycles. Simply notice your breath flowing in and out at the tip of your nose. Not adjusting your breathing, just allowing it to flow naturally.

o Find the place in your body where you are most clearly experiencing negative thoughts and feelings about a recent event or something that has been weighing on your mind. Often people feel sensations in their chest or belly area, but it can happen anywhere – just tune in to find yours.

o Simply breathe and be with that place in your body. Not trying to change it but merely cradling that space with loving, kind awareness, breathing in and out, staying there for several breaths and then returning to the room and opening your eyes. Thank yourself for paying loving, kind attention to yourself.

o This is an additional, more advanced, step you can try adding on once you are comfortable with the above:

– While cradling the feeling in your body simultaneously expand your consciousness outwards to the sounds in the room.

– Then take your mind outwards to the roof, the tops of the trees and continue expanding and broadening your consciousness, while continuing to return to and briefly touching the feeling in your body.

– Bounce back and forth between your expanded consciousness and feelings. When you are ready, return to the room – take your time to come back to your surroundings and open your eyes.

CLARITY &
CREATIVITY

UNLEASH YOUR CREATIVITY AND COLOUR THE WORLD

Just as you can influence the flow of your breath, so can your breath help you move through creative blocks and ignite seeds of inspiration. Creativity can be found in the most unlikely places and just like exercising your breath, you can exercise your creativity muscles by being open to seeing different perspectives, even within the mundane.

Being creative can mean taking risks and facing fears of putting yourself out there. Creating can feel agonising and excruciating because you risk failing and can't always see the outcome. Ideas can be spinning around with a map of spiralling routes which require space, engagement, exploration and trust to find the destination. Conscious breathing helps expand your inspiration while keeping those ideas grounded. When in the present moment, you unleash creative focus on ideas, making problem solving easier. When creative sparks fly, you feel more motivated, when ideas flow it creates more motivation and energy, and you get little hits of dopamine (see pages 167–171). This is the achievement hormone and the higher the dopamine levels in your body, the higher your alertness, focus, creativity, long-term memory and concentration.

When making the decision to step back and breathe mindfully you give the mind space to gain perspective, you choose to be in the present moment and that this is worthy of your full attention. Rather than escaping your busy mind, you can observe any turbulent thought patterns and by observing them you are no longer in them. You are the observer and you have a choice to stay there or move through without judgement, paving the way to opening other doors in the mind. By letting go and not pushing or putting a timeline on creativity, you take away the stress and deadlines. Creativity is a dichotomy of silence and noise, movement and stillness. Creativity only turns into a battle when the mind is overwhelmed, distracted, over-ambitious or lethargic.

EXPAND YOUR CREATIVITY

This short breathing exercise is designed to inspire your creativity. Think about your aspirations and dreams. When you breathe fully, you are inviting your psyche to be open to all of life's gifts.

o Place one hand on your heart and one hand on your belly. Close your eyes and take a few deep breaths.

o As you breathe quietly, notice the warmth of your hands on your belly and heart.

o Now, begin to breathe with the following intention:

Inhale. Breathe in inspiration. Exhale. I am in the flow and letting go.

Inhale. Breathe in expansion. Exhale. I am in the flow and letting go.

o Surrender to your breath and how you are feeling. Your creativity is limitless and knows no bounds.

o Inhale into your hand resting on your belly and then inhale into the hand on your chest. Gently release the exhale. Repeat.

o The inhale is two beats, starting with the movement in your belly and then up to your chest. Exhale and gently let go.

○ Continue this for a few rounds.

○ Expand your awareness. Let go of any thoughts. Relax and let go with each exhale. Where does your breath want to take you today?

Journaling

Journaling is a great tool to help creative flow. It increases self-awareness and your ability to process thoughts, ideas and feelings while freeing up space in the mind. When practising daily, you can notice patterns, behaviours and times when you feel more inspired.

Some women find they are more creative in the middle of their menstrual cycle and notice they have a creative flow at different phases of the moon (see more in Cycles, pages 269–290). You may find you get better ideas when out on a walk or run, or at different times of the day.

Write down your goals, what you are grateful for, what you feel limits you and what you would like to change. Notice your breathing when you put pen to paper and breathe softly. Research published in the journal *Psychological Science* shows that writing by hand has many more benefits than writing notes on your laptop or tablet. Scientists tested how taking notes impacts learning, and you have a better chance of remembering something if you take your time writing it down by hand. Research also shows that when you type on your laptop or on another device, you usually write down more, but end up remembering less.

Whether it's to write about life events, feelings or to explore your creativity, carry a journal with you and have one by your bed for those 5 a.m. epiphanies. Make journaling a

ritual and do it every day. By performing a breathing
exercise or simply being present with your breath for ten
minutes before you journal, you will find you are more open
and the inner critic is quieter.

HA BREATH

This exercise helps release blocks in the mind and body and activates the fire in your belly for inspiration. We often think of creativity as a flow of energy. Yogis say that when the energy moves upwards and passes through your centre, it's easier to access your subconscious and ignite your creativity.

o Stand with your feet shoulder-width apart and your knees bent.

o Place your hands on your lower abdomen and inhale through your mouth, making a loud 'Ha' sound from your throat to your belly on the exhale. Repeat this a few times.

o Raise your hands in the air and inhale. Clasp your hands together.

o Fall forwards with your hands still clasped and as you fall forwards loudly express the sound 'HA'. Then raise your hands up in the air and repeat this rapidly ten times.

o Notice how you feel.

Breathing with intention

When using conscious breathing exercises it is beneficial to set intentions for what you would like to achieve, such as creativity or having more clarity or focus. Try to make the intention positive and avoid negative words such as 'letting go of anxiety' or 'fear'. If that is what you would like to achieve, try not to focus on these negative words, but imagine letting go of them and how that will create space for creativity or clarity.

By focusing on the breath, letting go of any thoughts and paying attention to the rhythm of your inhale and exhale, you bring yourself back into the moment. It's easier said than done, but with regular practice it becomes easier and more achievable. By moving your focus away from your overthinking mind, you create space for creativity to flow. Often messages or insights can come after breathing exercises, somewhere totally random. Perhaps you'll be on a walk, cooking or a run when inspiration comes.

I recommend practising breathing exercises with intentions every day. Whether it's for one minute or five, you will notice a difference. It's not unusual to feel unfocused or lose your way at times. Setting intentions and practising dynamic rolling breathing exercises helps you to centre yourself. And if you can't think of an intention, that's OK too. Just set an intention to simply stay present with each breath. Here are some examples to inspire you:

'What do I want to let go of?'

'What would be meaningful for me today?'

'What action do I need to take in order to feel comfortable in my skin?'

'How do I want to feel today?'

'What energy do I want to feel, no matter what happens in my day?'

'If something is unresolved
and you can't see an answer,
your breath can help you to
become the observer, taking
yourself out of the story and
offering a different
perspective.'

CONSCIOUS CONNECTED ROLLING
BREATH WITH AN INTENTION OR PURPOSE

Find a time in the day that works for you to do this exercise. Some people find it easier first thing in the morning, while others prefer last thing at night. Play with it and see what suits you. Maintaining a daily practice and making it habitual will help you to fully feel the shifts and benefits. There will be times when five minutes feels like it's flown by and other times when it feels like an hour. Try not to be disheartened if you are more distracted from one day to the next.

- You can do this exercise sitting up or lying down. If lying down, bend your knees so your feet are flat on the floor. This will help your breath to come into your belly. Place your hands on your lower abdominals to help guide the movement there.

- Take a deep breath, bringing your focus from your mind to your heart space. Visualise your attention dropping into this space and take a few deep breaths.

- Ask, 'What do I need right now?' Then wait for the first word(s) that come up. Try not to overthink this. Consider what you would like to let go of, perhaps something that is holding you back. How would it make you feel if you could let it go? What would it bring more of into your life?

- If you want to let go of negative thoughts and feel clearer, your intention could be 'clarity.' Breathe in through your nose and relax your jaw.

LET IT GO

o Begin to breathe in and out through your nose.
  Emphasise the inhale and release the exhale gently;
  imagine you are misting a mirror with your breath. The
  exhale is effortless. Not pushing it out, forcing it out or
  hanging on to it.

o Repeat this and then connect the inhale to the exhale.
  There is no pause between the inhale and exhale.

o You may feel different emotions and sensations in
  your body. You may find you get hot or cold. Just allow
  any feelings and sensations and simply breathe
  through them.

o Your breath becomes one continuous circular breath.
  This may feel quite hard at first and your mind might be
  saying: 'But I have made a long inhale so I need to
  match the length with the exhale.'

o The natural mechanism of the exhale is to let go. Allow
  your breath to roll. A rolling breath with no pause. The
  breath always begins in the belly and moves up to
  the chest.

o If this feels too difficult, start breathing with your belly on
  the floor and making a pillow for your head with your
  hands. Connect your breath through your nose with no
  pause while lying on the floor. Once you feel the breath
  moving in your belly, roll on to your back with your feet
  flat on the floor and knees bent.

o After a few minutes, come back to your normal
  breathing pattern and breathe in through your nose.

Stay with this for another minute or two. Notice how you feel – more energised? Calmer?

o Finish with a big inhale through your nose and let it go with a big sigh out of your mouth. Repeat this three times.

Creativity in the workplace

Google recently looked at what makes the best-performing teams and the answer was everybody having an equal turn in conversation, with no one shutting others down, and an appreciation of different opinions. By forming this culture, creativity flourishes without hierarchy, the team explores skillsets and is flexible and able to innovate in an ever-changing world. If everyone is open and interested, people feel heard and not threatened by judgement. Performance is higher because the whole team feel respected, motivated and safe in their workplace.

The old strategies of playing people off against each other, giving negative feedback followed by positive, with silences in between, is similar to setting up a parent/child dynamic or being back in the playground. By working in a more fluid and less linear way, with gentle authority, the old patterns of hierarchy and wanting to control everything and everyone are no longer required.

CREATING SPACE FOR
CREATIVITY IN A GROUP

Often we can be in the workplace together but not all present, with our thoughts scattered and our minds elsewhere. Here's a very simple exercise to help let go of mind clutter to create room for clarity and calm. This is an exercise you can adapt for the beginning of a meeting for everyone to practise together.

Firstly, encourage the group to leave all thoughts at the door. Whatever it is they have to do today or tomorrow or should have done and perhaps haven't managed to yet, leave it all at the door.

○ Close your eyes and sit up straight.

○ Feel the ground beneath your feet and your sitting bones on the seat beneath you.

○ Relax and roll your shoulders back while letting out a deep sigh.

○ Begin to notice your breath and become aware of the inhale and the exhale.

○ Imagine your breath is coming in and out like a wave. Breathe softly and deeply in through your nose and out through your nose with a little pause in between.

○ As you inhale, guide your breath into your belly, encouraging a deep diaphragmatic breath.

o Allow your mind to wander to your breath and each time you notice you're going back to your thoughts, take your mind back to your breath.

o Begin to draw your focus and attention to the rise and fall of your breath. Allow the breath to flow. Not forcing it or pushing it. Just breathing gently.

o There is nowhere to go, nothing to do, just stay present with your breath. Everything is as it should be right now, there is no wrong and there is no right. Stay present with your inhale and your exhale.

o Notice any thoughts and gently push them aside. Step outside of the thoughts and observe them. Not entertaining them. Just allowing them to pass like clouds in the sky.

o Breathe in and breathe out, letting go of anything that no longer serves you. Exhaling away any tension or worries. Inhale in new energy, positivity and light. Let go of the pull of the future and the pull of the past.

o Continue to go deeper inside, explore and expand your awareness inside with each breath. Staying in this moment, which is NOW.

o Invite the group to stay with their breath, keeping their eyes closed and feeling their feet on the ground. After a couple of minutes, invite them to open their eyes. Notice the change of energy in the room.

Nature is your playground

All too often we neglect our greatest healer and inspiration – nature. If you're searching for creativity or overthinking, take yourself for a walk and the obstacle will seem less overwhelming. The beauty of getting outside in nature is that you start coming out of your head and connecting to your senses. Just walk and be, connect to your breath, stop the search, reignite your childhood wonder, use your imagination to turn nature into your playground and let creative thinking unfold.

In 2013, research published in the *British Journal of Sports Medicine* showed that walking in a city park or nature for as little as 25 minutes is enough to give your brain a rest and boost cognitive functioning. There was evidence of lower arousal, engagement and frustration, and of higher awareness when moving into the green-space zone; and of higher engagement when moving out of it. When the prefrontal cortex (the region of the brain involved in planning complex cognitive behaviour and decision-making) quietens down your overthinking mind it allows insight to come to you. It's akin to an 'imagination network'. It's activated when you're not focusing on anything specific and in a natural space such as a forest. The imagination network is absolutely critical to creativity. It draws on many regions across the brain, including the hippocampus, where memories are formed and stored, and the medial prefrontal cortex, which is involved in self-focused processing, including autobiographical memories. The imagination network is what enables us to envision other perspectives and scenarios, picture the future, remember the past, understand others and ourselves and create meaning from our experiences.

Whenever you feel overwhelmed or lacking ideas, simply take yourself off to sit under your favourite tree. If you are in the woods or in a park, tread quietly and listen, rather than think. Just breathe and be with the stillness.

WALKING MEDITATION

The next time you are struggling to find inspiration, instead of sitting in front of a screen, get out in nature. Give your brain a rest and boost cognitive functioning rather than waiting for the solution to come. Practise this exercise with a soft breath and an open heart.

o Take a walk somewhere in nature. If you live in a city, head to your favourite park or woodland area. Breathe through your nose.

o Before you begin, stand still, pause and put the rest of the day behind you. This time and space is for you. Turn off your phone.

o Feel the ground beneath you, take a few deep breaths, and become aware of your breath and notice where it is.

o As you walk at a normal pace, connect to your breath and take note of this constant companion that is with you throughout the day, feeling the rise and fall of your breath.

o As you place one foot on the ground and the other foot in front of it, notice how your feet feel and the change in balance as your body moves. Feel the constant connection to the ground with each step, allowing your arms to move freely, and become aware of the sights and sounds around you.

o Be here in this moment with each step, and every time the mind wanders, guide it back to the sensation of your feet on the ground, lifting, stepping, placing. Stay in the present moment.

o What colours and textures do you see? Have you spotted something you haven't noticed before?

o Take a few deep breaths and continue to walk at a gentle pace. Take your attention to the sounds around you: What do you hear? Focus on the sounds closest to you. Can you hear your feet on the ground beneath you, traffic close by, the sound of birds or people, the wind?

o Keep your attention on your breath and on the soles of your feet as you continue to move, and notice the rhythm of your breath, feeling peace and tranquillity with each step.

CONFIDENCE
&
SELF-WORTH

THE WAY YOU SPEAK TO
YOURSELF MATTERS

The pressure you put on yourself to be a certain way or
conform to societal expectations can sometimes leave
you feeling inadequate, separate or less than. To protect
and defend yourself against those feelings you can
subconsciously hold and limit your breath. Fear of failure
and making mistakes often prevents us moving forwards and
growing. Negative thoughts are like weeds that need
clearing so they don't take over the garden of your mind.
Instead focus on planting positive thoughts that turn into
beautiful flowers, tending them with love so that they
keep blossoming.

This doesn't mean you have to go around all day only
thinking positively and not feeling anything, but you do
have a choice in how you breathe, react and distract
yourself. The capacity to feel pleasurable emotions such as
joy, peace, creativity and a sense of belonging is directly
related to how well you acknowledge and allow
uncomfortable emotions such as anger, resentment,
shame or grief.

Perhaps there were times you didn't feel heard or seen. You may have had influences in life whose motivation was appearance or achieving results while not encouraging you to express more vulnerable emotions. Your parents may have been living vicariously through you by giving you a life they felt they didn't have. You may still be trying to get parental approval, and even though you have a list of successes or are a creative who is inspired moment to moment, it never feels enough. As you become more conscious of these patterns, you can make choices to align yourself with the here and now. Recognising being stuck in a loop of old programmes, past stories and belief systems helps you to better understand if you are reacting as opposed to responding to any given situation.

Be more tree

Trees don't judge each other and you probably don't judge trees. They are a good reminder to stay grounded, connect to your roots, drink plenty of water, be content with your uniqueness and enjoy the view. Showing your vulnerability can feel risky and you may feel that you will be rejected, misunderstood or turned away. When your inner critic is telling you 'This isn't good enough' or 'You're not intelligent enough', ask your inner nurturer to step in as your ally. Become a witness to the voices in your head and have compassion for them but know that they are simply voices and you have the power to turn the volume up or down.

Children are born with a spontaneous and carefree imagination. Stories transport you to wild and faraway places, being anyone you choose to be. As you grow, you become more aware of surroundings and cultural expectations, noticing how to fit in with different groups. The mind and body are equipped to create complex coping mechanisms to disguise social awkwardness and feelings of disconnect from others or the world around you. Being authentic should feel as natural as the sun setting and the seasons changing, yet if I asked you 'Who are you?' and 'What do you love about yourself?' how would you answer? Would you start with your job description and your marital status? These are labels rather than who you truly are. Ask yourself:

Who are you beyond the identities, the jobs and the mask?

What three things do you love about yourself?

HARNESSING YOUR POWER

By simply changing how you move or stand, you can boost your confidence and feel strong and powerful in your body. Psychological research suggests that postures and gestures affect psychological states and attitudes. Manipulating your posture can affect your thoughts and feelings.

o Stand with your feet hip-width apart, your spine straight and shoulders back. Visualise the top of your head with a thread pulling it up towards the sky. Your feet have roots grounding you into the earth.

o Tune into your breath and place your hands on your belly. Inhale into your hands, expanding your belly and contracting on the exhale for a few breaths.

o Bend your knees slightly and gently bounce. Close your eyes or soften your focus. Continue to bounce and allow your arms to fall by your sides. Feel your feet on the ground and keep your spine straight.

o Start to shake your hands and arms as you bounce and keep your breath slow and mindful. Do this for as long as you feel. Imagine letting go of any pent-up or nervous energy.

o Come back to a standing position and bring your hands into prayer position in front of your chest. As you inhale, stretch your arms out wide and as you exhale bring them back into prayer position. Imagine this is opening up your heart centre, chest and throat, letting go of any tension held here.

○ After a few rounds, come back to standing with your arms by your sides. On the inhale, raise your arms above you and on the exhale pull them down making a 'HAAAA' sound. This should be an energetic transition – as you are bringing your arms down remember to smile and feel the power in each 'HAAAA'.

○ After a few rounds keeping your eyes closed, take a few breaths into your belly with your hands resting on your lower abdominals and notice how you feel.

MICHELLE'S STORY

I met Michelle Barocchi at a gathering in Ibiza and we have since become great friends. She tragically lost her leg in a motorbike accident three years before we met and it was 40°C where we were staying with a lot of steep hills to climb. She went up and down them faster than any of us and while we were dripping with sweat, she remained a vision of utter beauty and confidence. We met in a breathing session I was holding and it was a powerful experience for us both. Michelle is a scientist specialising in immunology and also teaches yoga, breathwork and meditation. A predominant part of her teaching is to love and appreciate the body you live in and to find light in all the lessons that life teaches us. This is her story.

My breath saved my life on two occasions.

It was 11 August 2015 – I was riding on the back of a Vespa, rolling through the hills of southern Italy. We turned left and if it had been just a few seconds later, I might still have my left leg. The impact of the bright blue Fiat Punto tore through my body with the most exquisitely pure pain. 'Ahhhhhhhhhhhh,' was the primordial sound that expressed itself through my lungs and my vocal cords. I found myself thrown two metres to the side of the road, on my back, my helmet still attached to the side of my head. I thought: my life is over. Instead, my life had just begun.

The sky seemed softer and lighter. 'BREATHE!' said the voice I heard rushing through my veins. In that instant, my leg throbbing with pain, blood everywhere, I gasped for air,

147

and I knew I had less than five minutes to find a tourniquet for my leg or I would die. My intuition was spot on. Something was very wrong. I could see my left foot dangling, turned backwards in the most unfamiliar configuration for a human body. Something is wrong. I'm dying. I looked into my partner's eyes, holding the back of my left thigh. I could feel my breath soften; the golden hues of the sky were ever more subtle. I was numb.

I started to breathe a powerful breath I learned at a yoga teacher training course during the last few months of my doctoral training in Infectious Disease Immunology at UC Berkeley. *Ujjayi*, the breath of the warrior. A slight restriction of the throat allows for a sound to evolve through the breath so that the mind can focus, a technique of breathing meditation yogis have been using for centuries. I began to deepen and lengthen my breath and focused on the sound of the ocean in my throat.

In an instant, my partner Francesco and the other driver ran to call for help, and I was left alone with the sound of my breath and the sky. The air passing through my lungs was the air keeping me alive – the air of the sky. I was slowly becoming one with the sky. The sky was dissolving into me. Like the sky, I became silent. The sky is everywhere and nowhere, just as we accept our own silence – and in this silence we become the sky.

Help arrived with a crew of medics in an ambulance from Matera, and a helicopter landed in a field. I could feel warm fluid in my veins, and as they lifted me into the helicopter the medic gave me a thumbs up – keep breathing, come on, we're gonna make it. I woke up three days later from a pharmacologically induced coma with a new story.

Fast forward to July 2017, nearly two years after the event that changed the course of my life. A small gathering of indigenous elders came together for the first time to pray as a collective. It was there that I met the power of breath for the second time: Rebecca Dennis was sharing her knowledge of the power of breathwork.

After several minutes of conscious connected breathing, I was suddenly back on that road in Italy. Excruciating pain in my leg; total fear, rage and sadness embodied my entire being. I started shaking and then felt Rebecca guide me through an incredibly vivid and painful journey which ended in her holding me in her arms like a small child. My eyes were soaked with tears and as I looked around the circle, I realised I was not the only one. This was one of the most powerful experiences of my life. I was not new to experiences with higher consciousness and elevated dimensions, as I had been studying with Shamans in Peru for several years. But this was different. Exogenous forces mediate those experiences. This was mediated by my breath! I was empty. Empty of rage, of sadness, of pain, of judgement, and heavy emotions, which I had not been able to express since the amputation of my leg.

I currently use my scientific knowledge to study the breath and have joined my 20 years of yoga experience with my knowledge of Peruvian sacred practices to co-create journeys for people interested in uncovering their truth. My journey over the past five years since my 'accident' has taken me through a process of 'unlearning', teaching me how to remove the blocks I was holding on to and into the awareness of love's presence. There are many lessons I have learned through this transition; a transformation that has occurred on a physical level, but also a deeper transformation of my identity. Who I thought I was had been based on limiting beliefs. And what I know now is based on experience. I am not my body – as a recent amputee, I find that I have had to change my perception of the physical form of my body. As a human being, I was led to believe that I was whole because I had two arms and two legs, and therefore since now I have one leg and two arms, I am somehow 'not whole'.

I thought this was true because my mind attached itself to the belief that I was my body. But in order to evolve on the spiritual level, we have to become no-body. I have since learned that freedom (from attachment, from thought, and from pain) can only come when we understand that we are not our bodies, because the physical body is the limit. The physical body is purely a vehicle in which to express our pure essence, our energy. My leg is gone, but I still feel its energetic presence and this is what helps me move about on this earth.

If you don't get to know fear, you will never get to experience fearlessness. Fear is part of our life and growth. It's a big process of shedding old patterns. We have a choice to live as an expression of love or an expression of fear, and every breath we take will manifest one of these energies. So when you are in fear, just turn your head to the sun, and keep turning your head towards the light – keep choosing love, and breathe.

THE LIGHT OF THE SUN

Traditionally in yoga, control and expansion of life force (known in yoga as prana) was performed through reciting mantras. The breath was always practised with mantras in order to generate specific frequencies and vibrations in the mind-body connection. This exercise draws inspiration from those yogic teachings and uses the light of the sun and mantras together to boost self-assurance.

○ Sit in a comfortable position.

○ Place your right hand on your heart and your left hand on your lower belly. Take a few deep free-flowing breaths (at least three).

○ Inhale to a count of 4-3-2-1 into your lower belly – hold for a count of 2–4, visualising the light of the sun in your belly. Exhale, moving the energy up to your heart centre, to the count of 4-3-2-1, and hold for a count of 2–4 .Visualise the light of the sun in your heart centre.

○ Once you have practised this movement, you can (mentally) add the mantra 'om suryaya namah' either at the exhale or on both the inhale and exhale.

○ Repeat 12 times. Lie down for five minutes and enjoy the benefits of the sun in your body.

BUILD YOUR BOUNDARIES

Most of us have experienced insecurity. You can find yourself in a battle with the mind, anxiety and self-blame muddying the way you view yourself and the actions you take. The amygdala, part of the in-built alarm system in the brain, can prevent you from trusting your gut feelings or cause you to freeze in confronting situations familiar from the past. The good news is that your breath can help you strengthen your boundaries and each time a situation comes up it's an opportunity to clear old patterns.

'You can help your brain
to understand you don't
need to activate your worry
alarm system by moving
your focus to your breath.'

What you give power to, has power over you if you allow it. Naturally you want to please and be liked but you can't please everyone. You may feel lacking in self-worth and confidence because you have a partner, friend or colleague who infers you are never enough to match their expectations. If someone is making you feel that something is not right for you, then maybe it's time to let some people or patterns go, say no or decide you need to be in a working environment that raises and inspires you.

That friend, lover or parent can also be the internal voice in your head, giving you a hard time. When these thoughts begin to flood in, take a deep breath and come back into your body. You can help your brain to understand you don't need to activate your worry alarm system by moving your focus to your breath. You are enough. Be kind and full of compassion but know your boundaries. You may find yourself drawn back into people-pleasing patterns, seeking approval and seeing people who make you feel less than, saying 'yes' when you actually mean 'no'. Be your own voice and accept you can't please everyone. So cherish all the memories, but find yourself letting go and moving on. If you're currently dealing with this process you may feel a bit awkward, and that's OK. There will never be a time when life is simple. There will always be time to practise accepting that. Every moment is a chance to let go and feel peace with that.

HUMMING OR BEE BREATH

You can feel a shift in energy and more vibrant after humming for even just a minute or two. When you hum, you slow your breath and heart rate. The soft vibrations can help lull the vocal cords before a presentation or speaking. Toning or humming with your mouth closed has many benefits including improving stress levels, increasing lymphatic circulation, releasing endorphins and nitric oxide, which is fundamental to health and wellbeing.

○ Find a comfortable position with your spine straight and sitting bones beneath you. Lower your chin slightly without slouching your body forward. Keep your shoulders relaxed and chest open. Use your thumb or fingers to gently close your ears.

○ Relax your jaw and face. Close your eyes. Close your mouth, keeping your teeth slightly apart. Settle into the breath. Smile.

○ Inhale deeply through your nose and on the exhale create a slow, steady humming sound while visualising it moving from your throat down to the bottom of your spine.

○ Pause and take a few breaths into the belly using these affirmations:

'I am enough.'

'I am perfect as I am.'

'I am strong and I am powerful.'

'I am loving and accepting who I am.'

o Continue this for a few rounds. Notice how this makes
you feel.

SELF-LOVE

Self-worth is moulded from a very early stage and can take years of unravelling. How can we teach the next generation to love themselves for who they are and allow them to flourish and develop their own unique individuality? We need to start with ourselves by practising compassion and kindness every day. Children observe and mimic their elders. Monitor your screen time, love the body you are in and let go of the judgement of others. If you want children to believe they can be anyone they want to be, believe that you can too. Having a clearer understanding of what your boundaries are and how much you allow yourself to receive and express love in a healthy way can help children to feel safe and confident to express this also. There is nothing more beautiful than a person that knows their worth, loves the skin they are in and is in tune with their power and owns it.

Do you love the body you live in? Do you give yourself a hard time in the mirror? Is it easier to find fault with your body rather than seeing the parts that you love? Take a moment to just acknowledge how incredible your body is. Here you are living in this miraculous body with trillions of cells and neurons busy doing their work collecting information and keeping you running. The human body has its own ecosystem perfectly designed to keep you alive. However, when putting extra stress on it, your home doesn't feel quite so supportive and you start to berate and judge perceived imperfections, and tension accumulates.

Many memories live in your body, tissues and cells. Every emotion, comment and experience is recorded like data. When you consciously breathe into your body with intention, you are consciously connecting back into your home. Your body is your home.

You can feel safe in your home.

You can feel grateful for your home.

You can feel strength in your foundations.

Know it's your sanctuary and you can feel at peace here.

Yet sometimes you are ashamed of your home.

You get frustrated with its cracks and imperfections.

Some of the rooms in your home have not been visited for a long time, there are dust and cobwebs in subconscious doorways and possibly some ghosts. So how can you bring air and light back into all of these rooms and love the house you live in? Breathe life into each room. Stop yourself from giving it a hard time for not being the perfect house and nurture it with kindness instead. Breathe into your body, the body you live in and allow each breath to be a little love note to every part of you.

14-DAY FORGIVENESS

Inspired by the Hawaiian practice of Ho'oponopono, an ancient prayer that encourages forgiveness and acceptance of self to create space for healing, this exercise is most effective when it is practiced over a few days and it only takes a few minutes.

You're only as beautiful as you feel and that has to come from the inside first. This exercise helps reprogramme your thoughts, focusing on what you value rather than criticising and comparing yourself. Some days it's easier to find what you appreciate, like or love. It may feel uncomfortable and awkward but try this for the full 14 days and notice the difference.

○ Close your eyes and rather than judging and criticising, allow your mind to gently receive the image of yourself, breathing as you do. Notice how this feels. You are just witnessing your feelings. Take a deep breath in and softly and slowly release the breath.

○ If an inner conversation starts, such as 'Oh, I'm not good enough' or 'I can't control my thoughts . . .' bring your attention back to your breath. Keep your focus there. Simply letting yourself know 'I love you'. In the same way that you ingest food, ingest these words.

○ Begin to enquire with compassion into any negative beliefs. You may find that you feel sad as you bring more awareness to how you speak to yourself.

○ Recite these words 10–20 times and take a breath in between each line and feel the words entering every part of your being:

'I am sorry.'

'I love you.'

'Please forgive me.'

'Thank you.'

○ Once you have come to a point where you feel you are ready to close this exercise, take a breath in and out loud say: 'I love you'. If this is too much, try: 'I am learning to love you'. As you say this, smile with love and appreciation for your courage and where you are in this moment.

21-DAY SELF-CONFIDENCE BREATH

Coping with anxiety and low self-esteem isn't easy, but sometimes it helps to pause and reframe negative thought patterns while focusing on your breath. Practise this exercise for ten minutes every morning for 21 days. You can put on some background music to help connect to the rhythm and flow. After two tracks you will have done around ten minutes. If you miss a day, go back to day one. Keep the time and place the same so the exercise becomes habitual. This is not one to practise when you are feeling anxious but to practise daily so that any anxiety dissipates more easily during the day as you have set yourself up to feel confident and grounded.

o Sit upright in a comfortable position. Breathe into your belly for three or four counts and exhale slowly through your nose.

o Feel your feet on the ground and clasp your hands together in your lap. Bring your focus to your hands and feel them resting there.

o Take another breath in through your nose, visualising the breath coming all the way to the base of your spine and back up again. Keep breathing in and letting go.

o Count the breath in for four and exhale for a count of four for a few rounds and when you inhale use the affirmations. On the exhale allow the words to settle in:

'I am enough.'

'I am confident and powerful.'

'I am feeling grounded and calm.'

'I am perfect as I am.'

- You can write a journal after you've finished the exercise and record what you are feeling.

HAPPINESS & CONTENTMENT

BEING THANKFUL IS THE NEW MINDFUL

Happiness starts from within and taking time to notice and
appreciate what we have rather than what we don't have
is an often-recommended way to increase feelings of
contentment and positivity. The act of practising gratitude
is proven to enhance mental and physical wellbeing,
reduce stress, make us more inclined to join in activities
and look after ourselves. Yet some of the stuff that fills our
days such as deadlines and bills can get in the way.
Therein lies the challenge. Finding contentment in the
mundane and staying grateful even in the chaos.

'We are so busy doing, we
often forget how ordinary yet
extraordinary and sacred the
breath and life is.'

Go slow and appreciate where you are in your journey even if it's not where you want to be. Remember every now and then to let go, create space and pause. Breathe and become aware of all the beauty penetrating the corners of your life right now. So many of us are in a hurry to get to a future where we no longer need to hurry. We are so busy doing, we often forget how ordinary yet extraordinary and sacred the breath and life is. The air that we breathe is the same air that our ancestors breathed. It connects us to life and the rest of life on Earth.

So many of us live in a perpetual state of wanting more – more money, more shiny new toys yet sometimes slowing down and reflecting is just what is required to reconnect, get grounded and bring back perspective. When you choose to stop fixating on what you don't have and stop comparing and despairing you feel more inspired and satisfied with what you already have. And once you stop chasing happiness, you might just find that it appears naturally of its own accord.

An attitude of gratitude

Hebb's Law states that neurons that fire together wire together. The more times neural pathways are activated, the less time it takes to stimulate the pathways for the neurons to wire together. If we keep feeding our brain negative thoughts, the neural pathways for negative thinking become more stimulated. Practising gratitude sends positive messages to your brain via neural pathways and the more you stimulate these positive pathways, the more positive thinking becomes second nature. UCLA neuroscience researcher Alex Korb gives some insights that can help you to bring gratitude and happiness into your life:

'Everything is interconnected. Gratitude improves sleep. Sleep reduces pain. Reduced pain improves your mood. Improved mood reduces anxiety, which improves focus and planning.

Focus and planning helps with decision making. Decision making further reduces anxiety and improves enjoyment.

Enjoyment gives you more to be grateful for, which keeps that loop of the upward spiral going. Enjoyment also makes it more likely you'll exercise and be social, which, in turn, will make you happier.'

GRATITUDE BREATH

When you take the time to focus on your breath and the things you are grateful for the brain's 'bliss' centre releases dopamine and serotonin, generating feelings of joy and contentment. This exercise takes just a few minutes, so try it every day for a week. You can practise it lying or sitting and you can do it anywhere – in bed, in the shower, on the train or during a break at work. If you want to get the most out of it, keep a notebook handy to jot down what you are grateful for. Or keep a gratitude jar and write what you are grateful for on a piece of paper and put it in the jar. Try to write one or two things every day. See how you feel by the end of the week and carry that positive energy with you.

- Soften your focus and feel the ground beneath you. Allow your body to let go and relax your jaw, neck, back and legs.

- Take a deep breath in slowly and let the exhale go with a big sigh, releasing any tension. Imagine your breath coming into the top of your head and visualise an iridescent white light filling you with healing light. Feel it nourishing every part of you; thank all the cells in your body.

- Take a deep inhale, breathing into all the tiny muscles around your eyes, mouth and face, releasing any tension held here. Breathe into your neck and shoulders and on the exhale feel yourself letting go of any tension.

o Breathe into your arms and forearms, your wrists, hands and fingers. With each breath, send gratitude to all these parts of your body, visualising a white healing light filling these parts of you.

o Now breathe into your chest and ribcage. Take a deep breath into your heart area and thank your heart for beating every day and night. Let it know that you will treat it with great tenderness and care. Visualise breathing into all your organs, every vein, bone and muscle and imagine the iridescent white light filling every part of you. Send gratitude to all these parts of your body.

o Imagine your breath creating space in your belly, hips and thighs, sending gratitude with each breath. The white healing light is flooding down and coming into your legs, knees, calves, feet and toes.

o Each breath fills you with love for your body. Breathe into your whole body using the affirmation: 'I arrive in my body,' and when breathing out, affirm: 'I am home.'

o Breathe in through your nose and out through your nose. Make a long inhale and a little pause followed by a relaxed exhale.

o Feel your belly and ribcage expand as you inhale and contract as you exhale. As you breathe in, close your eyes and focus on three things you are grateful for. It may be your friends, the air you breathe, the sea, forests, a child's smile or a hug from someone you love. You might want to thank your body for working every day for you.

o As you breathe, feel energy coming into your body, healing your body, filling your cells and every part of your being. Stay with the rhythm of your breath, focus on every inhale and exhale and allow your breath to flow. Now feel that energy coming into all the people around you and the people you love. Feel them being healed and having the life they deserve.

OTHER WAYS TO GET YOUR DOSE OF HAPPY HORMONES

Dopamine	Oxytocin
Complete one thing on your list	Love
Book time off for you	Hug
Turn your phone off and watch the moon	Be kind
Help someone in need	Hold hands
Celebrate wins	Give someone a gift

Serotonin	Endorphins
Meditate	Breathe deeply
Run	Hug a tree
Spend time in nature	Laugh
Swim in the ocean	Dance
Practise gratitude	Listen to music

Dopamine – Also known as the 'feel-good' hormone, dopamine is a neurotransmitter that's an important part of your brain's reward system. Dopamine is associated with pleasurable sensations, along with learning, memory and motor system function.

Serotonin – This hormone (and neurotransmitter) helps regulate your mood as well as your sleep, appetite, digestion, learning ability and memory.

Oxytocin – Often called the 'love hormone', oxytocin is essential for childbirth, breastfeeding and parent-child bonding. It can also promote trust, empathy and bonding in relationships; oxytocin levels generally increase with physical affection.

Endorphins – Endorphins are your body's natural pain reliever, produced in response to stress or discomfort. Endorphin levels also tend to increase when you engage in reward-producing activities, such as eating or exercising.

THE COMPLETE BREATH

This exercise is great for shifting the mood if you're feeling a bit stuck in your head and you need to slow down your thoughts. Practise this exercise with a smile on your face and notice the shift in how you feel both physically and mentally after a few rounds. It engages your abdominal muscles and diaphragm instead of the upper chest and neck muscles, allowing more air exchange to occur in the lower lungs. This deep breathing allows higher volumes of oxygen to reach your body's cells and tissues, inducing feelings of release and calm.

o Stand up straight with your arms by your sides and your feet about a foot apart. Relax your body, jaw and shoulders.

o Feel your feet flat on the ground. Soften your focus. Gently push your abdominals out as you inhale through your nose for a count of five and lift your arms.

o Hold for a count of five, relax into the hold, then slowly exhale through your nose, contracting the belly and lowering your arms.

o At the end of the exhalation, pull your abdominals in and up which will push stale air from the base of your lungs. Hold your breath for four counts. Then push your abdominals out and inhale again.

o Repeat ten times and as you become accomplished, gradually increase the count to ten.

LISTEN TO YOUR GUT AND BE KIND TO YOUR HEART

The heart is an intelligent organ and when you feel calm and balanced, your heart rate is rhythmic and slow. When you experience fear, excitement, stress or anxiety, these emotions change the rhythm of your heart. The breath is there to bring the balance back. Consistently showing up, allowing yourself to be vulnerable and authentic is the route to refining your relationship with yourself and others. When you can be open to love while knowing you may also experience feelings such as grief and pain and sadness because it's all part of life's rich tapestry, you dare to life live more fully. When you cut yourself off from pain because of past hurt, you also cut yourself off from experiencing other emotions such as deep joy and ecstasy.

There is growing evidence to support the link between the gut and our mental health. There is a constant two-way communication between the brain and gut called the gut-brain axis and so stress can have a direct impact on your gut. Diaphragmatic breathing helps the digestive system work more efficiently by stimulating the rest and digest state (PNS response, see page 27) and helping you let go of any tension you may be holding in your core. It's good to remind ourselves that the gut carries millions of neurons communicating messages via the nervous system to the brain. A happy gut = a happy mind. An incredible 70% of your serotonin (see page 170) is produced in your gut, so by breathing into and internally massaging this space, you are actively improving your 'gut feeling'. What you feed your gut is not just what you eat; it's what you watch, listen to, read, the people you surround yourself with, your lifestyle and thoughts and most importantly, how you breathe.

DIGEST AND BREATHE

Great for any time, especially bedtime.

○ Lie down and relax your whole body. Place your hands on your belly, let your inhale push your belly up into your hands, allowing the stomach to relax. Take about 15 deep belly breaths.

○ Turn to the left side gently and fold your knees. Place your left hand under your head, right hand on your right leg and adjust your posture to be comfortable.

○ Lying in this position, inhale and exhale 21 times consciously and count the numbers. When on your left side, your stomach gets compressed to the floor and internal massage is happening inside the abdomen, helping digestion.

○ Come on to your back with your legs stretched out and place your hands on your belly again. Raise your hands on the inhale and exhale, relaxing your hands back down by your sides, mentally counting 21 breaths.

○ Repeat on the opposite side.

JESS'S STORY

I am very lucky to have some magical people in my life and Jess Horn is one of them. Jess is a yoga and meditation teacher, making it accessible to everyone no matter where they are on their yoga journey. She shares some wise words on happiness below.

I've explored many different tools and techniques for over 20 years, taught by masters from all different walks of life, and I've learned that the most healing are those that give us the ability to find balance, develop resilience and feel centred when life knocks us off course. For me, the most powerful tools are those that give us time to experience stillness and silence in order to connect to our inner space.

Many of us feel like we are always 'on' and due to technology have a sense of always being available and needing to answer questions constantly, with the division between 'home' and 'work' increasingly blurred. Where before there would have been more naturally occurring moments of stillness, now we have to make a conscious decision to practise it. We don't spend time daydreaming on the train or walking without sound, company or music. Even in our showers or baths we are often listening to podcasts, music or books. We are constantly trying to be productive, to learn more and we end up filling all of the silent spaces. I believe it's never been more important to cultivate the ability to 'do nothing' by performing exercises where we rest in stillness, presence and silence.

We are in an age where we are constantly bombarded by noise and information. I have over seven different ways that people can contact me and often people expect near instant replies. Everywhere I go there is music, radio, TV, mobile phones, podcasts, stimulation for our already overstimulated brains and for many of us it's actually become addictive and the prospect of being on our own in silence is very daunting and challenging. It's worth experiencing the discomfort though as there is so much healing in the absence of noise.

The real beauty and power is what occurs when you begin to experience the inner peace and stillness that is naturally there within. It's within this stillness that you can begin to listen to your heart and inner wisdom rather than being ruled by the often irrational and sometimes mean inner voice of ego! In silence and stillness, you can begin to experience the infinite nature of your being, which is spacious, loving and peaceful. It's been shown that when we give ourselves time to daydream, to be, we are more creative and productive.

FINDING HAPPINESS THROUGH
STILLNESS, SPACE AND SILENCE

The practice of doing nothing, looking inwards rather than outwards, befriending yourself and being comfortable with your own company without distractions, noise or places to hide is not always easy, but it's definitely rewarding and can help you develop self-acceptance. In time you'll begin to feel less busy, less easily distracted and more joyful, just through the practice of doing nothing!

o Start with a walk in nature, on your own and without your phone – no headphones, just you and your lovely self. At first it might feel awkward, but stay with it. I promise you there is more joy there and you'll be more in the moment and feel refreshed in your mind as well as your body.

o When you're in the car, don't automatically switch on music or the radio but invite in moments for stillness and reflection.

o Take a bath with no music or sounds to hide behind – just you, your body and your breath.

o As this becomes easier, begin to sit for a few minutes every day in stillness, observing your breath and thoughts, watching the natural pauses that eventually might build up into velvety moments of bliss and peace. Remember you're not trying to still your thoughts or push them away, rather become the observer and practise surrendering thoughts as they arise, returning to your breath and the pauses in between.

Maybe over time this might develop into a regular meditation practice, the benefits of which are huge, but maybe it's as simple as ensuring you carve out little pockets of silent space throughout your day so you can learn to be happy without needing anything or anyone. The important thing is to give yourself time just to be, to experience silence and the stillness of pauses between breaths and thoughts which eventually can lead you to a feeling of infinite SPACE and JOY.

ENERGY

ENERGY EVERY DAY

A lot of us are looking for that 'boost' of energy – indeed it might be why you have turned to this very chapter for an alternative to a quick sugar or caffeine fix. There are breathing exercises you can access much quicker than a coffee or chocolate bar, for free, without any of the nasty come-downs afterwards. Some of the exercises here can be used when you hit that 4 p.m. crash or you've slumped and need energy for a meeting at the end of a long working day or helping the children with their homework. There are also long-term strategies for improving your everyday energy levels, which counterintuitively mean slowing down to achieve balance, so you're not constantly on an energy roller-coaster, where highs are followed by inevitable lows.

Most cultures, in one way or another, acknowledge the existence of a life-force energy. 'Spiritus' comes from Latin meaning 'to breathe', in Sanskrit it is called 'prana', in China it is 'chi' and the Japanese call it 'ki'. 'Prana' and 'chi' mean both 'energy' and 'breath' because you can generate energy by practising breathing exercises. When you work with your breath, you create energy to process lower vibrational emotions such as anger, sadness, anxiety and create space for inspiration, clarity and motivation. We often live from the shoulders upwards and spending too much time in your mind can disconnect you from how you feel in your body, but by combining movement with your breath, you can plug straight back in and raise your vibrations. Here's a really simple, high energy-inducing exercise to try.

DANCE BREATH

Inspired by Kundalini yoga, which originated in India and focusses on meditation that is believed to fully awaken your awareness, this is a great exercise to do with family or on your own – practise it first thing in the morning or whenever you hit an energy slump. It's particularly effective for releasing tension from long sedentary days, while allowing pent-up emotions to escape the body and mind.

o Find your favourite dance track (optional) and begin to gently bounce up and down with your feet on the ground, moving your hips and bending your knees, or if you feel more energetic jumping up and down.

o Stand with your feet shoulder-width apart and knees bent.

o Raise both arms above your head as you inhale through your mouth.

o Exhale through your mouth, as you bring your arms down with your elbows in towards your ribcage and your hands to shoulder height. Inhale through your mouth.

o Inhale as you raise the arms and exhale as you bring them down.

o Repeat for two minutes at a moderate pace and increase time and intensity as you progress.

ENERGY IS EVERYWHERE!

Everything in the universe is made up of energetic molecules vibrating at different speeds – trees, stones, water, your body, thoughts and emotions. In simple terms, some molecules vibrate fast and some vibrate more slowly; there are higher vibrations and lower vibrations. Research has shown that your thoughts and behaviours affect the rhythms and chemical reactions in your body. For example, anxious thoughts trigger the release of stress hormones that stimulate your heart to speed up or slow down. The sound vibrations of music, likewise, affect your mood, emotions and bodily functions. We all can feel emotions, such as joy, peace and acceptance, creating high-frequency vibrations making us feel lighter and happier, while other feelings, such as anger, depression and fear, vibrate at a lower rate making us feel heavy or low. If you are depressed, your breath may feel laboured or shallow, when you are excited or nervous your breath will become more rapid and fast.

The Law of Entrainment states if two vibrations of different frequencies vibrate together then the higher vibration will lift the lower one to meet it. So when you consciously connect to your breath, otherwise known as your prana or life-force energy, you begin to raise your vibrations and start to move physical tension and emotional blocks. When you are present in the moment, you are not in the past or future, you are in the flow of life. Conscious breathing calms your nervous system and brings about greater feelings of connection. The time has come for you to raise your vibrational forces!

GET HIGH ON YOUR OWN SUPPLY

This rolling or wheel breath is a real energiser and a game changer if you're feeling stuck or lacklustre. It's also a good hangover cure as it stimulates the lymphatic and digestive systems to help detox the body. By stimulating both the sympathetic nervous system and parasympathetic nervous system you lightly increase adrenaline which causes more glucose to be available in your bloodstream for your body to burn as fuel. This technique acts as a pendulum, stimulating energy while also inducing feelings of calm.

You can practise this sitting up or lying down; try to find a space where you won't be interrupted.

o If you are lying down, bend your knees so your feet are flat on the floor. This will help the breath movement to come into your belly.

o Place one hand on your lower abdominals and the other hand on your chest. Breathe slowly and mindfully into the hand on your belly. Allow the inhale to push your belly away and on the exhale, contract.

o Set an intention for this exercise. Think about what you would like to let in. How would that make you feel and what would it bring more of into your life? Maybe there is something you want to change in the way you think or feel.

o Breathe in through your nose and out through your nose. Relax your jaw.

o Emphasise the inhale and relax the exhale. Not pushing the exhale out, forcing it or hanging on to it. Let it be a soft, relaxed, gentle sigh.

o Repeat and then connect the inhale with the exhale. There is no pause between the inhale and exhale. Inhale into the hand on your belly and then inhale into the hand on your chest and then let go on the exhale. Not blowing the exhale out, just gently letting go.

o Allow your breath to become one continuous circular breath. This may feel hard at first and your mind might be saying, 'I can't do this'. Allow your mind to follow your breath. Be aware of any feelings or sensations and simply be with them and breathe. Remember active inhale, passive exhale.

o Start to move your arms, either pounding them on the ground or punching them in the air and moving your legs like you are running on the spot. Make some sound like an 'Ahhhhh' or an 'Ooooooooooo', and then come back to the circular breath and place your hands back on your belly and chest.

o Feel and notice the shift, and the opening and expansion of your breath.

o After 2–5 minutes, return to your normal breathing pattern and breathe in through your nose. Stay there for a while and allow your whole body to let go.

o Notice the subtle movement of the rise and fall of your breath. Notice how you feel, perhaps more energised or calm and clear.

o Finish with a long inhale through your nose and let it go with a big sigh out through your mouth. Repeat three times.

Tips: Remember to relax the exhale. The more you practise, the more it will flow with ease. If it ever becomes overwhelming or you can't get the movement of the breath into your belly, just slow your breath down or turn on to your tummy face down until you can feel the breath pushing your lower abdominals away.

LIFE IS TOO PRECIOUS TO HACK

We all know that quick fixes are generally too good to be true. More often than not, they're a temporary solution to any root cause. Healing and letting go of that which isn't serving you takes different amounts of time for different people and comes from allowing space and time to step back from overwhelm to accept and respect where you are right now. While expending your energy on a quest for immediate results, it makes it harder to see how far you have come and to be content with what you already possess. The more noise drowns out your intuitive abilities, the more susceptible you are to being cajoled by promises of fast tracking and achieving 'superhuman' results.

With so much advice out there, over-stimulated minds skim read and share information and research from overnight experts or memes. While technology is in many ways extraordinary and ground breaking, it moves us further away from our connection to nature and our natural ability to read and listen to our own bodies and minds. It may seem counterintuitive in a world that is addicted to speed, but the slower you move, the faster you heal and learn to trust your own inner compass.

The pursuit of wellness is swiftly developing into another million-dollar industry with promises of inner calm, looking forever young and reaching higher states of awareness. But with this pursuit, we risk devaluing the idea that life is there to be fully felt, to experience the messy, incredible, awful, inspirational and uncomfortable. You can be vulnerable and still powerful – life's true lessons come from experiencing both the ups and the downs. Space is everything, perspective is everything. So take a moment to check in, breathe and remember who you were before life got to you.

THE FIVE RITES OF REJUVENATION

The Five Rites consist of five movement exercises and are reported to have been created by Tibetan monks over 2,500 years ago. I have adapted these movements with particular focus on breathwork, drawing inspiration from the booklet *Ancient Secret of the Fountain of Youth* by Peter Kelder, who introduced this concept to Western culture. According to the booklet, the lamas of India describe seven spinning 'psychic vortexes' within the body: two in the brain, one at the base of the throat, one on the right side of the body near the liver, one in the reproductive anatomy, and one in each knee. As we grow older, the spin rate of the vortexes diminishes, resulting in 'ill-health'. However, the spin rate of these vortexes can be restored by performing the Five Rites daily, resulting in improved health.

This sequence will stretch and strengthen your body. I recommend starting with 3–5 repetitions of each movement and then adding one repetition each day, building up to a maximum of 21 repetitions.

LET IT GO

Rite 1

Move slowly and mindfully, working with your breath. Don't look at this as a vigorous exercise, but as a way to energise and bring balance to your body.

o Stand up straight with your legs hip-width apart.

o Extend your arms to the sides at shoulder level, with your right palm facing downwards and your left palm facing up.

o Before you start spinning, pick a spot in front of you to focus on every time you turn.

o Breathe deeply and slowly through your nose while spinning from the right and keeping your feet in an imaginary circle. Stop if you start feeling dizzy.

o Once you have completed the turns, centre yourself by placing your hands in prayer position and stay with your breath.

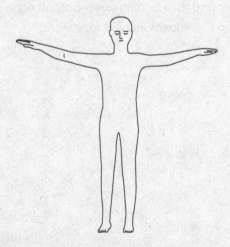

Rite 2

This might be a more familiar exercise; it strengthens your legs, lower back and abdominals as well as massaging your organs to help your digestive system function well.

○ Lie on your back with your arms next to you, palms facing down. Inhale as you raise your head off the floor, tucking your chin into your chest. Simultaneously lift your legs into a perpendicular position. Exhale while slowly lowering your head and legs. Repeat, lifting your legs and head off the ground simultaneously. Every inhale: raise your legs and head; every exhale: lower your legs and head.

Tips: To make this easier, bend your legs until you get strong and flexible enough to straighten them. It also helps to place your hands underneath your buttocks to support your lower back. Focus on engaging your muscles consciously on the way up and down.

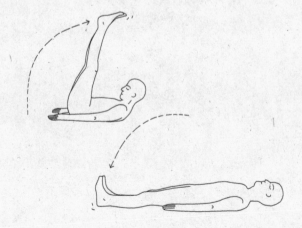

Rite 3

This can look similar to camel pose in yoga. It is good for stretching your stomach and intestines, improving flexibility of the spine and stimulating the nervous system.

o Kneel on the floor with your arms alongside your body and palms on the back of your thighs. Curl your toes underneath your feet, or lay your feet flat on the floor. Draw your shoulders away from your ears and start with a deep inhale. Hold your lower body still.

o Inhale, and rotate your shoulders backwards and squeeze your shoulder blades together. Reach your arms around and place your hands under your thighs.

o Press in your hands while curving your head back with your gaze towards the sky. Relax your lower spine and only bend from your upper back.

○ Exhale as you come forwards. Softly drop your chin to
your chest. Every inhale: move backwards. Every exhale:
come forwards.

Tips: Avoid forcing the movement with your neck and
follow the weight of your head. Do the exercise slowly so
you don't put any unnecessary pressure on your spine
and neck.

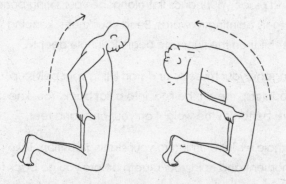

Rite 4

This exercise requires arm, leg and glute strength to do it correctly, as well as some wrist and neck flexibility. This rite is said to help the digestive, nervous, respiratory and lymphatic systems and fire up the glutes.

o Sit on the floor, legs stretched out in front of you and back straight. Leave some space between your legs and place your hands flat alongside your sitting bones, fingers pointing forwards. Bend your knees, keeping your feet flat on the floor and begin to inhale deeply.

o Engage your muscles and start lifting your pelvis up. Let your torso rise off the floor into a flat back. Your knees are bent with the weight on your arms and feet.

o Exhale while returning to your starting position. Take a moment and hold your breath before you go back to lift up again. Every inhale: raise off the ground. Every exhale: return to your starting position.

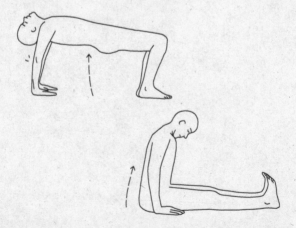

Rite 5

You may be familiar with yoga moves downward dog and upward facing dog. This final exercise involves doing both in a steady and flowing motion. It is good for alleviating lower back tension and helps circulation.

o Lie flat on your belly with your hands next to your chest as if you were about to do a press-up, but with your elbows against your body.

o Inhale deeply and press yourself up by straightening your arms, opening your chest and curving your back. Your legs are straight, shoulders down and away from your ears. Look up by drawing your head back slightly. Start exhaling when lifting your hips up and back into the air. Elongate your spine and drop your heels as far back into the floor as possible. Rest your head by looking at your knees.

o Repeat in a flowing motion. Every inhale: downward facing dog. Every exhale: upward facing dog.

Tips: If you are not very flexible, you can slightly bend your knees.

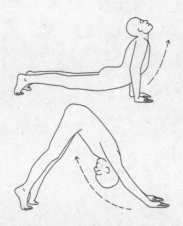

SLEEP

REST. RESTORE. RESET.

Children have a lot of energy but they also get a lot of sleep! As adults we are not always good parents to ourselves and few of us follow a routine to induce good-quality sleep. While we are all increasingly aware of the importance of getting a good night's shut-eye, many of us scrape by on a few hours, while worrying about not getting enough.

Good sleep is conducive to a feeling of wellbeing. When your sleep suffers, you don't just see bags under your eyes. Lack of sleep has serious effects on your brain's ability to function. If you've ever pulled an all-nighter or been burning the candle at both ends, you'll be only too familiar with the side effects – grumpiness, irritability, mind fog and forgetfulness. Sleep can affect your focus, your weight and even how you age; it isn't just a stress-reliever for your mind and body, but your skin too. Lack of sleep increases your cortisol levels, putting your skin in a pro-inflammatory state, as well as increasing your risk of obesity and type 2 diabetes as key hormones which play a role in weight gain and controlling appetite are released during the night.

With insomnia rising at an alarming rate, sleep is considered a luxury rather than a necessity that we require to regenerate, heal and recharge. When you sleep your brain goes into repair mode; sleep is linked to memory, learning and the mechanisms of neural plasticity. A healthy amount of sleep is vital for brain plasticity, or your brain's ability to adapt to input. If you sleep too little, you become unable to process what you've learned during the day and you have more trouble remembering it in the future. Researchers also believe that sleep may promote the removal of waste products from brain cells – something that seems to occur less efficiently when the brain is awake.

Sleep has been traditionally divided into four categories: awake, light, deep and REM (Rapid Eye Movement). Each one plays an essential role in maintaining your mental and physical health. During non-REM sleep (about 80% of an adult's sleeping time), you breathe slowly and regularly. But during REM sleep, your breathing rate goes up again. That's the time we typically dream. Breathing also becomes more shallow and less regular during this sleep phase. REM sleep is important to your sleep cycle because it stimulates the areas of your brain essential in learning and making or retaining memories. Deep sleep is when the pituitary gland secretes important hormones, like human growth hormone, leading to the growth and development of the body. If you are worrying or fretful it is harder to reach those deep sleep stages for the required time to restore and rejuvenate.

RITUALS FOR SLEEP

Try committing to little rituals before you go to bed so your body and brain know that you are winding down ready for a restful and restorative night's sleep.

- Have a warm bath with candles, lavender and Epsom salts. Practising a few minutes of gentle belly breathing in the bath helps to stimulate the parasympathetic nervous system (see page 15). A good place to have five minutes' peace from family or other household members as well.

- Make yourself a mug of warm 'golden milk' with a mugful of milk, some turmeric, a little ginger, black pepper and a teaspoon of honey. Turmeric is believed to help reduce inflammation in the body, aid your liver to detoxify, boost your immune system and ease your digestive system – all of which help you get to sleep faster, sleep better and wake up feeling refreshed.

- Read a book in bed or listen to calming music rather than watching another episode on Netflix.

- Try magnesium supplements – studies show that people with magnesium deficiency often have issues sleeping. Use as flakes in the bath, as a spray or as a dietary supplement.

- Enjoy essential oils in a diffuser in your bedroom – lavender, chamomile, clary sage and frankincense are all relaxing and calming fragrances.

- Remember to unplug your phone or put it on airplane mode and try to keep screens out of the bedroom so it's a space solely for rest and relaxation.

Two-thirds of UK adults suffer from disrupted sleep patterns, while nearly a quarter manage no more than five hours a night. Increasing pressure to perform, pay the bills and other daily challenges can lead to long periods awake at night. It's tempting to embrace bad habits and use stimulants like sugar, alcohol, caffeine, pharmaceutical drugs and recreational substances to stay awake or help you unwind. Research suggests that more than one in ten people take sleeping tablets or drink alcohol to aid sleep, but instead of turning to substances, try looking to your breath to help you fall asleep or get back to sleep if you wake in the night (see next page).

4-7-8 TECHNIQUE

This breathing exercise can help you feel calm if you wake up at 2 a.m. with a busy mind, and stimulate the nervous system into a relaxed state. By focusing on counting, your mind is distracted from busy thoughts and eventually gets bored into sleep.

- Lie down in a comfortable position and close your eyes. Press the tip of your tongue to the roof of your mouth. Slightly open your mouth and exhale until you reach the end of your breath.

- Close your mouth and quietly inhale through your nose for four counts. Hold your breath for seven counts. Exhale slowly and gently through your mouth for eight counts.

- Repeat for four full breaths, working your way up to eight breaths over time.

MINI YOGA NIDRA

Yoga nidra is a deeply restorative practice originating in
India. Its roots can be traced back to philosophical writings
recorded around 700 BC. When your mind is busy, go
through the following exercise and you may find you fall
asleep before you reach the end. You can find a longer
recorded version of this in my podcasts of free guided
breathing exercises *And Breathe*.

o Lie on your back on a bed, with your arms and legs
   outstretched. Find a comfortable position, with your
   palms facing up and your legs wider than hip distance
   apart. Make sure you're covered up and comfortable,
   and that you won't be disturbed, in case you do fall
   asleep!

o Become aware of the position you are in. Feel the
   imprint of your body on the bed. Allow your body to
   become heavy and fully supported by the bed. Know
   you have nowhere to go, nothing to do. Become aware
   of your breath, you don't need to change it or do
   anything to it, just become aware of it coming in and
   going out. Feel where your breath moves your body as
   you breathe. Notice your belly rise and fall, a gentle
   sense of expansion with your inhale and softening and
   relaxing with your inhale.

o Bring awareness to your right hand, thumb, first finger,
   second, third, fourth. The palm of your hand, back of
   your hand, wrist, elbow, upper arm, shoulder, armpit,
   side body, right hip, thigh, knee, calf, ankle, heel, sole of

the foot, top of your foot, right big toe, second toe,
third, fourth and fifth.

o Bring awareness to your left hand, thumb, first finger,
second, third, fourth, palm of your hand, back of your
hand, wrist, elbow, upper arm, shoulder, armpit, side
body, left hip, thigh, knee, calf, ankle, heel, sole of the
foot, top of your foot, left big toe, second toe, third,
fourth and fifth.

o Bring awareness to the back of your head, back of your
neck, right shoulder blade, left shoulder blade, spine,
right buttock, left buttock.

o Bring awareness to your forehead, feel the skin on your
forehead relax, feel your right eyebrow, left eyebrow
and skin between the eyebrows relax. Right eye, left
eye, feel the eyes relax within their sockets. Feel the right
cheek and left cheek relax. Feel your nose, left nostril,
right nostril relax. Feel your mouth, top lip, bottom lip,
even the space between your lips relax. Feel your
tongue, the root of the tongue, following your
awareness down your throat to your chest. Feel your
right side relax, then your left side. Feel your upper belly,
feel your lower belly. Imagine all of your organs relaxing.

o Bring awareness to your whole body deeply relax.
Become aware of your breath again, just following the
inhale and the exhale, the rise and the fall of the belly.
Count backwards following the inhale and exhale:
inhale 21, exhale 21, inhale 20, exhale 20, inhale 19,
exhale 19, inhale 18, exhale 18, inhale 17 . . . etc.
Continue down to zero. If you lose count, start again

at 21.Take a long pause. Stop counting but keep your awareness on the gentle ebb and flow of your breath. Feel that with every exhale your body is becoming a little heavier and a little stiller and that with every exhale sleep is coming your way. Stay aware of the softening of your breath, notice how gentle it becomes.

LEGS UP DIAPHRAGMATIC BREATHING

By relaxing your body, it becomes easier to relax your nervous system, which sends messages to your brain that you are setting the stage for restful sleep. Add some gentle breathing and the effects are even better. This exercise also alleviates menstrual cramps and helps to relieve swollen ankles and varicose veins. It's a good stretch for the back of the neck, front torso and back of the legs and gently boosts blood circulation towards your upper body and head, which creates a lovely rebalancing after you have been standing or sitting for a long time. Practise this restorative pose at night before getting into bed.

o Lie down and bring your sitting bones close to a wall by gently raising your legs up against the wall. Your sitting bones don't need to be right against the wall, depending on the tightness of your hamstrings. Place a pillow underneath your head and allow your shoulders to relax. Coming into this pose may take practice. Experiment with the position until you find the placement that works for you. Soften your jaw, face and shoulders.

o When you breathe in, your diaphragm flattens downwards creating a vacuum that draws in air. When you exhale, it returns to its dome shape, pushing air out of your body. Rest your hands on your lower belly so you can feel your breath expanding. Breathe in slowly through your nose. Let the air flow as you inhale and expand your belly – expanding your sides and lower ribs, filling your diaphragm, back and lower back. Allow the deep inhale to push your belly out.

○ Let your breath go with a gentle sigh through your nose or mouth and feel your belly coming in. Don't force the air out – simply allow it to flow in and out of your body.

○ Keep your legs relatively firm, just enough to hold them vertically in place. If you struggle to keep your legs upright, take a yoga strap or something similar and place it around your legs just below the knees, then gently tighten to hold the legs upright, allowing you to relax further into the position. Stay in the pose for 5–20 minutes, allowing your breath to return to normal for the last few minutes. When you are ready to come out of it, bend your knees halfway towards your chest and roll to one side. Use your arms to help you sit up, moving slowly and mindfully.

SLEEP APNOEA AND SNORING

Breathing through your mouth when you're asleep can cause you to wake up feeling groggy with a dry mouth, which also affects dental health and stress levels. Long-term mouth breathing during sleep and sleep apnoea are also associated with high blood pressure, cardiovascular and metabolic issues and even dementia. If you currently suffer from other breathing-related sleep disorders, it is very likely that you are a night-time mouth-breather.

Mouth taping has proven to be successful for many cases and people report feeling more energised when waking. Please consult your doctor before you practise this and never cover your whole mouth with tape. I'd recommend practising during the day first before trying it out at night. A small strip will do and use a light tape such as surgical tape, not gaffer tape! Patrick McKeown, author of *The Oxygen Advantage*, advises using Myotape. This does not cover the mouth but surrounds it, bringing the lips together with a light, elastic tension that helps to maintain lip closure and ensure nasal breathing. This elastic tension serves as a continuous reminder to keep your lips together.

If you find yourself waking up without mouth tape despite sticking it securely the night before, it is a fairly accurate indicator that you are indeed a recurrent mouth-breather! This might be due to a blocked nose, sinus infections or severe sleep apnoea, so do ensure that you treat the underlying problem before giving mouth taping another go and consult your GP first.

IMMUNITY &
RECOVERY

YOUR IMMUNE SYSTEM

The immune system is your body's front-line defence against viruses and infections. It acts as your housekeeper, tidying and cleaning the environment inside and monitoring the environment outside. The immune system is constantly processing information and accessing repair and maintenance needs, it isn't just about fighting off germs or disease. The communication between the immune, respiratory, digestive, endocrine and nervous systems affects your psychology as well as physiology.

The air you breathe converts into chemicals needed to fuel your cells. All cells need glucose and oxygen for respiration. Glucose is broken down into carbon dioxide and water and this makes energy available for the reactions which take place in those cells. Oxygen enables metabolism, the breakdown of dietary carbohydrates and fats which converts them into energy. The way you breathe affects your stress response, cortisol levels and blood pressure. Cortisol is the body's stress hormone and high levels are associated with autoimmune diseases, adrenal fatigue, poor sleep, hormone imbalance and promoting inflammation. So by using conscious breathing techniques to help deal with stress, you reduce your cortisol levels and improve your wellbeing. There is a free prescription to boost your immune system and it's right under your nose!

'Use your breath as a tool to guide you through challenging times, bring in balance and support your wellbeing.'

Breath-holding to strengthen your immune system

According to a study by the Norwegian University of Science & Technology, breath-holding doesn't just change the genetic activity of white blood cells. It also significantly increases the amount of white blood cells in the body available to help fight illnesses. For the purpose of the study, the researchers obtained blood samples from world-class divers at an international competition before and after the athletes completed a series of dives. The results were striking: the activity of more than 5,000 genes (almost a quarter of all genes found in human cells) changed in response to the simple effort of breath-holding. The most striking finding was a significant increase in the number of a specific white blood cell type: neutrophil granulocytes. These blood cells are programmed for rapid response when the body is under attack from infections and viruses.

DEEP BELLY BREATHS WITH BREATH HOLD

It's best to practise this exercise first thing in the morning or when your stomach is empty. Some days you may notice the breath hold is longer and easier than others. You may feel light-headed or dizzy when you begin this. It is perfectly safe and you can try it lying down to help any light-headedness.

o Find a comfortable seated position. Close your eyes and tune into your breath. Inhale deeply through your nose, then exhale without pushing or forcing through your mouth.

o Fully inhale through your belly, then chest and then let the breath go.

o Hold your breath by holding your nose on the inhale and start to roll your head back and forth and sideways for a few seconds. This helps to unblock the nose for nasal breathing. Repeat twice.

o Exhale and inhale again deeply and fully.

o Inhale and exhale in short powerful bursts 10–15 times, inhaling through your nose and exhaling through your mouth. At the bottom of the final exhale, close your mouth and hold your breath for as long as it feels comfortable. When your body wants to inhale, inhale and then exhale.

o Repeat the whole cycle 3–4 times.

Note: This is not advised if you are pregnant.

YOUR BIOGRAPHY IS IN YOUR BIOLOGY

Science has long established that thoughts and emotions have physiological consequences and not only are your cells storing data from your thoughts but you can build up your immune system through behavourial patterns, diet, lifestyle habits, exercise and conscious breathing techniques.

Dr Candace Pert, the neuroscientist and pharmacologist who discovered the opiate receptor, the cellular binding site for endorphins in the brain, explains how deep breathing can change your physiology, both clearing old emotions and balancing bodily systems. She says: 'Your subconscious mind is really your body. Neuropeptides are small molecules that brain neurons use to communicate with each other. The brain releases the neuropeptides in order to regulate physiological systems by communicating with receptor sites throughout the body. They carry emotion inducing chemicals to the receptor sites.'

Deepening or changing your rate of breathing is effective because the respiratory system is a concentrated location for receptor sites, including receptors for every kind of peptide the body uses. When you change the rate or depth of your breath, according to Dr Pert, it triggers the release of emotion-carrying peptides from the base of the brain. Neuropeptides include natural endorphins and opiates, which, aside from enhancing happiness, can relieve pain. This also begins to explain why for thousands of years sages and yogis have been able to use their breath to manipulate bodily functions such as blood pressure and heart rate.

In times of stress, your body releases more inflammatory chemicals. This starts a chemical cascade in your protection system and your body and brain have to try and work out what is required to stop an attack on your body. In fight-or-flight mode your body prioritises your muscles, cardiovascular and respiratory systems – the other systems, such as the immune system, are lower priority, so keeping stress under control is important for your long-term health.

Breathing to boost immunity and reduce anxiety

The nose is your first line of defence before air reaches your lungs and when you're feeling stressed, unwell or anxious your breathing is affected and you might catch yourself sighing or clenching your jaw. Not only does nose breathing regulate air from cold to warm before it reaches your lungs, but it also produces nitric oxide, which combats harmful viruses and bacteria while regulating your blood pressure.

The expansion and contraction of your diaphragm when you breathe stimulates your lymphatic system and acts to massage your internal organs; 60% of your lymph nodes are situated under the diaphragm. The lymphatic system works closely with the immune system to help the body extract and purge internal toxins.

FIGURE OF EIGHT BREATH

When you are feeling anxious there is a tendency to hold your breath, contract muscles or shallow breathe. Often when you're overwhelmed or in pain, your breath can feel stuck or laboured and it's harder to gather your thoughts. To help alleviate anxiety and support your immune system, try this very simple balance breathing technique.

o Inhale through your nose for four counts.

o Exhale through your nose for four counts. If this feels too hard, reduce it to three counts.

o Begin by using your breath to expand your lower abdominals on the inhale and contract on the exhale.

o Take slow gentle breaths in through your nose and out through your nose.

o Relax your shoulders and focus on your breath, moving your belly as you breathe.

o As you breathe in and out, visualise a figure of eight starting from the pelvis, travelling just above your belly button up to your chest and back around again. Continue this visualisation while gently following your breath.

o Continue for 1–2 minutes and practise at different times throughout the day.

TRUST YOUR GUT

Breathe deeply and learn to trust the voice of your gut. It's widely acknowledged that the gut is your second brain, so called because it develops from the same tissues as your central nervous system during foetal development. Even though the research is relatively new and complex, it is clear that the brain and gut are intimately connected. Given how closely the gut and brain interact, it has become clear that emotions can trigger symptoms in the gut and research has shown medical treatment can be less effective than holistic methods.

A pilot study from Harvard University found that meditation could have a significant impact for those with irritable bowel syndrome (IBS) and inflammatory bowel disease (IBD). Forty-eight patients with either IBS or IBD undertook a nine-week programme that included meditation training and the results showed reduced pain, improved symptoms, stress reduction, and even a change in expression of the genes that contribute to inflammation.

Further more, there is now research that is dubbing depression as an inflammatory disorder mediated by poor gut health. Multiple animal studies have shown that manipulating the gut microbiota in some way can produce behaviours related to anxiety and depression.

PILATES BALL
TO AID DIGESTION

Abdominal tension, alcohol, irritating foods or stress can slow the digestive system or even lead to irritable bowel syndrome. This abdominal massage technique generates movement in your belly, assisting the inner movement necessary for healthy gut function.

You can use a Pilates ball or roll up a medium-sized towel into a ball. Roll the towel lengthways first and then roll it the opposite way into a tight ball.

o Lie down flat, resting your belly on a Pilates ball or rolled up towel. Allow your head to rest on the floor with your hands by the sides of your head, palms down.

o Breathe into your belly and use the ball or towel to massage your abdominals. This can feel intense at first, so go at your own pace and stay there for around 2–3 minutes.

Note: This is not advised if you are pregnant.

CAT/COW

This is a practice regularly used in yoga and helps to relieve pressure in your lower back, stomach, chest and shoulders. It also helps to reduce bloating by stretching and contracting the abdomen.

○ Start in a tabletop position with your knees hip-width apart and arms shoulder-width apart.

○ As you inhale, raise your head and tailbone towards the ceiling, looking up as you bend your back.

○ As you exhale, curl the head in and tailbone down, creating an arch with your back.

○ Repeat 10–20 times, or as needed throughout the day.

SLOWING DOWN IS THE FASTEST WAY TO HEAL

When practising restorative breathing exercises, you allow your muscles to let go, trusting the ground to hold you completely, feeling into where you are holding any tension and letting go a little more with the next breath. This creates release and ease in the body, reminding you that it's not sustainable to keep working and doing without respite for repair.

When you're recovering from illness, burnout or an operation, it can take time to get your energy back and there may be a backlog of work, life commitments, calls and emails to answer. When experiencing stressful thoughts or pain, your breathing becomes shallow and primarily the breath movement comes from the upper chest. This can make you feel short of breath and hungry for air, prolonging the recovery period which brings on feelings of anxiousness or frustration.

As well as reversing the physical stress response in the body, restorative breathing can help repair your body while calming and slowing down the emotional turbulence in the mind. You switch over from worrying about staying 'safe' and not feeling pain to fostering the systems which support long-term health, including digestion, elimination, reproduction, growth and repair and immunity.

'Take a rest, a field that has rested gives a beautiful crop' Ovid

ABBIE'S STORY

When Abbie came to see me she was in debilitating pain. She worked in the world of TV for many years and was always comparing herself to others, never feeling her appearance was good enough. Desperate for perfection, she underwent breast augmentation surgery. Little did she know that this would be the demise of her physical and mental health and result in her being diagnosed with an incurable autoimmune condition. (This is now referred to as Breast Implant Illness (BII) and recognised by the MHRA and FDA.) Nearly four years on, Abbie's journey of healing through detoxing, diet and better breathing has kept her off strong medication and able to live life to the fullest.

In 2015 my whole world came crashing down when I was diagnosed with an autoimmune condition that left me bedridden at times and in a whole heap of pain. I felt my life as I knew it was over. I couldn't see any light at the end of the tunnel and I spent many hours on the internet searching for a magical cure. I struggled with the fact that this was how my life was going to be from now on. A life of pain, with the only option taking a chemotherapy drug weekly to suppress my immune system to stop it attacking itself, which had the side effect of making me hideously nauseous. My gut instinct told me not to give up and that eventually I would find the answer to why my body decided to flip out on itself and cause so much distress.

Trusting that instinct was undoubtedly the best thing I have ever done. It showed me that there was far more to the situation than I could have possibly realised. In my twenties I decided to have silicone breast implants. For years I had been complaining of exhaustion, hair loss, headaches and dizzy spells but because I was a new mum always on the go, I just put it down to my hectic lifestyle. It turns out that my implants were making me sick for 11 years and the final straw for my compromised body was my immune system falling apart.

As I set out to rectify my condition, I came up against a lot of negativity from my doctors and consultants who simply wouldn't believe that there was any correlation between my implants and autoimmune condition. This caused me immense stress and anxiety, mixed with confusion and utter panic that I was doing the right thing for my health. I cried most days, became more depressed and at times it led to very dark thoughts of taking my own life. With my body already in a vicious cycle of stressors due to the implants, this added pressure made my health even worse.

After finally removing the implants, it was the perfect opportunity for me to stop taking the chemo drug (against the advice of my rheumatologist) and start the process of detoxing my body to give it a fighting chance of healing. As well as receiving help from an amazing nutritionist who gave me huge insight into my gut health and how nasty microbes can cause imbalances and bring on autoimmune issues, I also came across breathwork with Rebecca. Working with the breath was the final piece of the puzzle for my journey. It handed me the tools I needed to still my mind, gave me the clarity I so desperately needed and calmed my sympathetic nervous system, allowing my body to realign itself.

The wonders of breath didn't stop there for me either. Due to the lack of exercise in my life, as I was feeling too rotten to do anything most of the time, my lymphatic system was unable to remove any bacteria, toxins or viruses. There was no real movement or contraction of muscles to make it flow and my normal breathing pattern was very shallow due to the pain I was in. Deep diaphragmatic breathing sessions gave my body gentle yet effective workouts that stimulated my very sluggish lymphatic system to do its job properly.

It is now six years since my journey back to health began and it has been one hell of a roller-coaster. With no information on how to heal from a set of silicone implants that cause your immune system to go AWOL, I had to find my way through the dark to the light, be my own doctor at times and trust my instincts. But my health has never been better. I haven't felt the need to go back on the chemo drug and each year I get stronger and stronger. There are still little blips every now and again, but these are nowhere near as intense as they were and they aren't happening as frequently. What is so wonderful is that when they do sneak up on me, I know exactly how to handle them because I have all these incredible tools to calm my mind, press the reset button and release any unwanted pain.

Breathing through pain

When experiencing pain, the body releases stress hormones, promoting inflammation and aggravating the pain. Breathing exercises help you reframe your focus and shift the nervous system which helps to reduce inflammation and pain. When in a quieter state of surrender through breathwork, your body isn't flooding itself with stress hormones. This is why women have intuitively known for centuries, or been told by their midwives, to work with their breath when in labour.

Focusing on your breath can help to release endorphins, which are natural pain relievers (see pages 170–171). Some days this will feel more effective than others but even by simply giving your mind another focus you can distract from the discomfort. The tissues and muscles around the pain centre are in a less contracted state when you feel calmer, helping to ease the source of the pain. Research in mindfulness-based stress reduction, which combines meditation and yoga, has shown it to be effective for alleviating chronic lower back pain and releasing tension around the body.

BODY SCAN

Body scanning involves paying attention to parts of your body in a gradual sequence from your feet to head, noticing any tension or general discomfort while allowing your focus to move to other areas where there is less pain. The aim is not to relieve the pain but to manage it and reduce stress and inflammation. Often emotional stress caused by pain can bring on further discomfort, such as headaches, back and shoulder pain and digestive issues. This body scan helps release tension you might not realise you have which, in itself, can reduce symptoms.

o Lie down on a bed or the floor. Make sure the room is warm and you are comfortable. Perhaps put a pillow under your knees.

o Take a deep breath in through your nose and out through your mouth.

o As you breathe out, close your eyes. Notice how your body feels.

o Starting at the top of your head, scan your face, eyes, ears, nose and mouth and then move to your throat, neck and shoulders.

o Slowly and mindfully scan down your body, noticing what feels comfortable and what feels uncomfortable.

o Your mind will wander and that's OK; it's about learning to recognise that your mind has wandered so you can bring your focus back to your body and your breath.

o Remember, you're not trying to change anything, just noticing how your body feels as you scan down and notice every part of your body.

o This can take 5 minutes or 45 minutes. Stay present with your breath and allow it to be slow, not forcing or pushing it.

ASTHMA AND RESPIRATORY ISSUES

Air pollution is critically high with asthma now one of the most common diseases. I regularly see clients with chronic asthma and respiratory issues and they tend to hold a large amount of tension in their diaphragms, which creates tension in the intercostal muscles (the muscles in between the ribs) and a feeling of tightness in the chest.

Asthma can be brought on by the environment, allergies or experiences that have not been fully processed. It can also be due to a combination of these factors and I like to play with the breath, see where the muscle tension is restricting the breath movement and look at how to release the tension that prevents the breath from flowing. When you find it difficult to breathe, it can cause anxiety and panic and the tendency is to breathe more up into the chest, causing gasping and increasing the hunger for air.

Many of my clients no longer have to use their inhalers as a result of this style of breathwork and while I can't promise you the same results, the exercise below is an excellent foundation to begin developing an open, healthy breath. Practising conscious connected breathing is also a very effective way to ease the symptoms of asthma and I recommend working with a trained breath coach when practising this first.

RELAXING EXERCISE FOR ASTHMATICS

It is advisable to always prop yourself up at a 45-degree angle when practising this type of breathwork if you have asthma. This helps to expand the space for lung capacity by freeing up the diaphragm and also opens your chest and shoulders.

o Sit on the floor with a cushion beneath you and lean your back against a wall. Alternatively, lie on the floor, making sure you are propped up at a 45-degree angle with cushions or pillows.

o Inhale a slow, deep breath through your nose.

o Place one or two fingers directly on the space just below your breastbone and apply gentle pressure. This is your solar plexus (see page 68) and may feel tender or tight at first due to accumulated tension – as you continue to breathe you will feel the tension and tenderness subside.

o Exhale freely, quickly and easily, as if you are releasing a big sigh.

o Consciously ask your body to relax. Feel your upper chest soften as you breathe. Keep your shoulders down and use your lower abdominals to expand in and out on the exhale. Relax completely while breathing in and out through your nose.

o Repeat for about five minutes while maintaining soft
and gentle breathing and acupressure. Don't be
discouraged if this doesn't happen immediately.
Remember that you are working with years of
unproductive patterns of breathing.

LUNG EMPTYING

This is a really useful exercise for asthmatics or anyone getting over a chest infection or prone to bronchitis. This technique helps to clear fluid from the lungs when recovering from an infection, but can also be done daily to help circulate the air in the lungs. This may bring up mucus, or cause you to cough deeply so it could be useful to have tissues handy.

o Take 3–4 deep breaths into your belly through your nose.

o At the end of the exhale, when your lungs feel empty, cough 3–4 times.

o Repeat twice more.

Note: If you have a pre-existing lung condition, go very gently. If it is severe, please only do this with supervision from your doctor. I do not recommend doing this forcefully if your lungs are inflamed as it can be painful and may irritate the lungs further.

Recovering from respiratory issues

When recovering from viruses or respiratory issues there can be weakness and damage to the lungs and respiratory system. With so many people affected by chest and respiratory issues we all know people struggling with their breathing. Practising regular breathing exercises can help improve the function of the diaphragm, get more air to the base of your lungs, reduce and generally improve the supply of oxygen to your lungs and body. A lot of fear and anxiety comes with feeling you can not get enough air. These exercises are simple and effective when practised regularly.

PURSED LIPS BREATH

When you're feeling breathless or have a tight chest from a cold or flu, this breathing technique can help you get the air you need without working so hard. Often when you've had flu or a chest infection you hold tension in the shoulders. Before you begin this exercise, take a moment to drop your shoulders down, soften your jaw, close your eyes and relax.

o Breathe in through your nose, as if you are smelling something, for about two seconds.

o Pucker your lips like you are ready to blow out candles on a birthday cake. Breathe out very slowly through pursed lips, making your exhale two to three times longer than your inhale.

o Repeat for a few rounds.

LUNG STRENGTHENING BREATH

Stretching exercises lengthen your muscles, increasing flexibility and exercising the lungs, helping to increase your overall lung capacity and elasticity. I recommend using this technique as part of a daily practice. It is especially good to do before other exercise, breathing exercises or meditation.

- Make sure you are sitting or lying down as breath holds may cause dizziness.

- Close your mouth and inhale through your nose until your lungs are full of air.

- Pause for three seconds and then take a sip more air through your nose.

- Pause for three seconds and take a second sip through your nose.

- Pause for three seconds, then let the air whoosh out through your mouth.

- Repeat twice.

Note: As this exercise includes breath holds that may cause dizziness, please go very gently. If you have epilepsy, high (or low) blood pressure or a history of fainting or stroke, please seek the advice of a medical professional before practising.

LUNG DRAINING

This is recommended by nurses working with patients experiencing breathing issues as an effective way to release mucus from the lungs.

○ Begin with long exhales with a 'Ffff' sound while blowing up your cheeks. This creates resistance to the outgoing breath so that the pressure on the lungs increases during the exhalation. This helps to inflate the alveoli, the smallest passageways of the lungs, activate the tissues and release mucus.

○ To increase the effect, lie on your belly, chest upside down (on a Pilates ball or some pillows), so that the mucus can flow easily out of your lungs. Additionally, if someone is with you, they can tap on the back of the lung area.

RIA'S STORY

Ria was diagnosed with cancer this year and is currently undergoing treatment. This is how her breath has helped her physically and emotionally through these tough times.

There have been times when life has taken my breath away: the birth of my daughter, the towering mountains surrounding Lake Wakatipu in New Zealand and being reunited with my family in Sydney. There have also been moments when life has felt suffocating, where I have gasped broken sentences between tears on hearing the words that create terror in many: 'Your cancer has returned.'

As the summer of 2020 hit, I became accustomed to holding my breath figuratively and literally, with the general anxiety of a pandemic alongside multiple scans, biopsies and consultations. My body was becoming a storage vessel for unexpressed emotions and a deficit of missed exhales. By autumn, I felt like I was falling into an abyss and when the news confirmed what I feared the most, I hit rock bottom. I had become lost in the fog and overwhelmed by the velocity of information that so many cancer patients experience. Amidst it all I had forgotten that a powerful force that would help me was also on the inside!

I experienced many dark nights of the soul during that period and each time I visited those places I became more familiar with the visceral and somatic experience. I could no longer contain the fear, terror and consequential strain of those emotions on my body and I started to find gaps in those experiences. Those gaps, thanks to both support from Rebecca and my daily meditation practice, allowed me to recall other supportive practices I have learned over the years. I knew that facing a life-threatening diagnosis would understandably create a pattern of fear and immense stress. It was time to be present with what arose and counter it with unrequited kindness, staying anchored to my breath to cultivate connection, calm and clarity.

From the moment I woke, my breath became a key part of my day. Creating space for breathing practices – meditation, yoga and conscious breathwork – allowed me to make friends with cancer and the emotional and mental landscape that goes with it. Throughout my life, I have suffered from panic attacks and chronic anxiety and Rebecca has supported me on the journey to healing my body, through connecting with my breath. It became a significant part of my treatment plan, alongside chemotherapy. The breath became my compassionate companion and a bridge between mind and body.

After five months, and towards the end of my chemotherapy, my energy levels plummeted and fatigue enveloped me. I had never felt such nausea, at times hopelessness and breathlessness. Before my final chemo cycle, I had the opportunity to join Rebecca for an online session focusing on yoga and breathwork. I was familiar with the techniques Rebecca was going to use and felt I needed the time with her to give me the fortitude to move towards this final cycle. A few weeks before the session, I was waking up each morning with a mouth like sandpaper because the soreness and stuffiness in my nose had become so awful that I was often only able to breathe in and out through my mouth. The session itself was a welcome break from lockdown, home schooling and weekly medical treatment. Being guided, cared for and supported gave relief to the tension I had been holding on to despite my practices. The familiar sensations I experienced during the session as I focused on my breath felt like they were reintegrating my mind, body and emotions. It was a much-needed reprieve and release of so much. When I woke the following morning I noticed my nose was clear, my mouth wasn't dry and I didn't feel sluggish. It emphasized how our breath can be our most faithful companion.

The lessons I am learning during my cancer treatment are opening my eyes to the opportunity every one of us has to have a deeper, kinder, more connected and subtle relationship with our amazing minds and bodies through the power of being present with our breath and each moment.

BREATHING FOR
POSITIVE HEALTH

Using affirmations with breathwork has a powerful effect on maintaining a healthy body and mindset. When you change the narrative, you reconfigure your neural pathways which triggers the nervous system to come out of fight-or-flight mode to support your immune system more efficiently. The more you practise this, the more those neural pathways fire together.

o Sit up or lie down. Tune in to your breath and breath in through your nose and out through your nose. Rather than the breath moving up and down visualise it moving in and out.

o As you breathe in and out use any of the following affirmations or create your own. Repeat 2–3 times:

'My immune system is strong.'

'My mind is focused on healing my body.'

'My mind and body are in perfect harmony.'

'I send positive energy to my immune system.'

'My immune system is strong.'

'I am starting to feel healthier and stronger.'

'My body is naturally resilient to pain.'

'I can recover quickly from any health problem.'

'I am breathing consciously and this keeps my immune system strong.'

'My mind is focused on healing my body.'

FAMILY &
CHILDREN

BREATHING EXERCISE FOR EVERYONE, EVERY DAY

It is essential for children and teenagers to be able to grow from their experiences – both negative and positive – and not shut themselves off from the world. Bullying and self-harm is escalating among boys and girls and the levels of anxiety, stress, depression and suicide are also rising in this generation. Gaining compassion for themselves and others helps children to respect cultural diversity, differences and understand their own body prejudices.

When you teach breathing exercises to children, you give them a life-long tool for managing their stress, boosting self-confidence, building resilience and cultivating inner peace. Integrating breathing exercises into their day at mealtimes, bedtime or on the way to school helps them to notice how different breathing exercises affect how they feel, think and respond to certain situations. By simply taking the time to pause and breathe consciously they can create healthy habits which become a way of being rather than something they are being told to do.

Just as you are taught to brush your teeth, tidy your room, bathe, communicate, say 'please' and 'thank you', it's also a good reminder that practising breath exercises is good for emotional and mental hygiene, helping to manage feelings and shift mind-body state. Families and children can use these tools of conscious breathing to help them manage and shift their feelings throughout the day.

Good times to practise breathing with the family:

In the morning to set a positive mindset for the day.

At night to wind down before sleep.

Before a big test or exam.

When struggling with anxiety, conflict or confidence. For managing emotional turmoil.

BREATHING THROUGH LIFE

One of the most important lessons we can teach children is how to use their breath as a tool for life. The transition from innocence to awareness and everything in between – shyness, fitting in, the desire to conform – is a complex one that can be navigated more consciously by using the breath. Often children find it hard to express their feelings or understand the turmoil of surging hormones and emotions, and everyone living with them can feel those moments! It's also important to note that most adults are still harbouring parts of their inner child that has not felt heard or seen, so this chapter is beneficial for everyone.

Breathing exercises can help you move through complex times. When you harness the power of conscious breathing and encourage children and young adults to explore their feelings, it creates ways for them to cultivate their inner wisdom and strength. When you experience unpleasant emotions or stress your body responds – you breathe faster or more shallowly, you may feel your cheeks burn or have knots in the stomach. Often when a child is experiencing anxiety or upset it can feel physical and come in the form of a headache, rash, feeling sick, nervous tics or stomach ache and the child or parent may not be aware that the physical reaction is in fact emotional. When you are finding it hard to verbalise your feelings, another route to connect to the inner world of turmoil and create calm is to sit with those feelings and use gentle safe touch and the breath.

HAND TRACING BREATH

This is an exercise all the family can do together or children can practise when in need of some time out or to feel calm. It's relaxing, easy to follow and great for emotional regulation. It can be practised anywhere sitting or standing.

o Fan out your fingers with your hand in the air, on your knee or a surface.

o Use the index finger of your other hand to begin tracing along the hand that is fanned out, starting from the thumb to the little finger.

o Inhale through your nose as you trace the outside of the thumb, then exhale through the mouth as you trace along the inside of your thumb.

o Inhale as you trace the outside of your index finger, exhale as you trace the inside of your index finger . . . and so on until all your fingers have been traced.

o Notice how the small movements feel.

o When you are finished, reflect on how you are feeling. Is there a difference in how you feel afterwards?

BEA'S STORY

Bea started coming to breathing sessions with me after experiencing chest pain and anxiety attacks. Through conscious connected breathing (see pages 230–232) she was able to feel the pain of her grief and other emotions attached to her story. Since working with me, Bea has attended and helped facilitate some group sessions; her story opens up the room for others to connect to their own inner child and give themselves permission to be vulnerable.

I was three when my dad left. My primary school made me feel 'othered' because all the families looked perfect, cereal packet families – the kind society suggests you should strive for. Both parents would come to the school play, harvest festival and the nativity. My mum would always be there too, cheering louder than anyone and supporting me. But I didn't see that; I saw what I didn't have and everyone else did: a dad, two parents, the 'perfect family'. I felt like I was unwanted, that I didn't fit in. Overwhelming emotions for a child.

Then I started secondary school. I instantly felt like I fitted in, almost everyone had a mismatched family. But that Christmas one of my close friends died. He was a beautiful, kind, caring person who would always think about others even when many mistreated him. This was my first proper encounter with death and it sent a wave of emotions through me. For the first time I cried for someone else I knew I would never get back, I longed to see him again and I had to deal with the fact that I couldn't.

The pain became so bad that it started to affect me physically. I frequently got a very tight feeling in my chest. Anything could bring this on – a teacher telling me off, forgetting to do my work or not catching the early bus (even though I knew the next one would still get me to school on time). These anxiety attacks became so bad that eventually Mum took me to A&E and I was rushed on to an ECG machine to check my heart. I physically couldn't breathe and it was so frightening. A twelve-year-old in hospital because I didn't know how to process the pain. The nurse eventually came to the conclusion that it was emotional.

My mum is friends with Rebecca and she booked me a session with her. At first it felt insanely weird, so many emotions and physical reactions from this intentional, repetitive breath. It was hard to stay with it but it really helped. As I came to more sessions, I began to feel more open to the idea of healing, of allowing myself to get better. Rebecca gave me the opportunity to tell my story at the beginning of her group sessions. I wrote what I wanted to say and read it out to about 50 people each time. The way the therapy works is she helps you to understand your pain, she helps you feel better about it, feel stronger. Like you are in control.

Over time I realised that I didn't want to forget the pain, because if you forget you lose a piece of who you are. A piece of your story. One of the puzzle pieces that makes up the complicated million-piece jigsaw puzzle that is you. So, I didn't forget, I tried instead to understand it and release it. That is what the power of breath helped me to do. The simple, repetitive, natural thing we do each day. The thing we can't stop doing because it is what keeps us going. It is the breath that changes when we see someone we love, when we get nervous, when we are happy. It is the repetitive flow that happens even when the rest of us is turned off. It is the thing that helps us become calm when we feel anxious or scared. It seems like such a small thing but when used with the intention of healing, it can cure decades of pain. And that is what it did! I haven't had those tight chest pains that caused me to not be able to breathe since. I haven't had the churning twist in my gut when something goes wrong. Breathing exercises helped me to reshape those puzzle pieces of my life so they fit just right, so that they no longer bring me down and so I can grow and still be me.

RESTORATIVE GROUNDING BREATH

When feeling overwhelmed, exhausted or finding it hard to gather your thoughts, this exercise helps you recalibrate and reset. It's deeply restorative and soothing for the nervous system and helps you to feel safe in your body. Great for teenagers when it's exam time and they may be finding it hard to focus or switch off, or for little (or big) ones before bedtime.

o Lie down on a yoga mat or soft rug, with your belly on the floor. Make a pillow for your forehead with your hands. Feel the support of the ground beneath you.

o Breathe into the ground by pushing your belly down on the inhale and letting go on the exhale. Visualise giving your energy to the ground beneath you and drawing energy back up from the earth to re-energise you.

o Imagine that you collapsed into the ground, like you simply had no more energy to give. Start feeling the physical sensations under you on the surface of your body. Feel the ground under your hands, forehead, chest, belly, pelvis, thighs, knees and feet. While feeling these sensations, feel the earth beneath you, cradling and supporting you.

o Keep your breath gently moving in and out through the nose and the movement in your belly and lower back.

o From your hands and knees, lower your hips toward your heels. Spread your knees apart (or they can be together) while feeling the tops of your feet on the ground. Extend your arms forwards with the palms of your hands flat on the floor. Rest your forehead on the floor and your upper body on your thighs.

o Feel your breath move in your belly into your thighs. Breathe in for a slow count of five, then breathe out for a slow count of five. Stay in this pose for as long as you wish.

o When you feel ready, come into a seated position with your spine straight and gently lean from one side to the other, putting your arm out to find support, then leaning to the other side. Feel the support under your hand, then lean away to the opposite side.

o Come back to centre, take a few breaths and notice how you feel.

ELLA'S STORY

I asked my friend and colleague Ella Oliver to share her wisdom on how breathing exercises can help young adults regulate their minds, bodies and emotions. Ella regularly holds workshops for teenagers called Puff and Glow.

Young people's wellbeing has changed significantly in the last 20 years. The pace of modern life, instant communication, exposure to comparison, social media, technology-centric communication in school life, shame culture, generational trauma plus the coronavirus pandemic has created a pressure cooker of unrelenting expectation on our next generations.

Adolescence is a period driven by self-discovery, exploration and trying to understand who we want to be in the world. It's also a crucial time to develop and maintain wellbeing and social, emotional habits that sustain us in an empowered and healthful way so that we can self-soothe and regulate our minds, bodies and emotions through the inevitable vicissitudes of life. The growth of mental health issues in young people has not happened in isolation and in order to understand the challenges they are facing we need to look at the world we have created.

The technological advancement we have been privileged to encounter means we are able to complete mundane tasks in a fraction of the time of previous generations, we connect immediately across borders, yet we often overlook that in order to achieve these seemingly impossible feats. We emphasize our intellectual prowess and favour the importance of brainpower in defining who we are and at the expense of other aspects of our humanness. We must remain aware of the need to balance out these intellectual progressions with our worlds of emotion, physical feedback, chemical and energetic reality. Our education systems are measured with a disproportionate bias towards intellectual and mental might, which moulds young people with expectations that value cerebral attainment and skill building above everything. This continual accentuation on the mind in part steers measurement of attainment and self-worth towards what young people's minds are producing and the need to perform well in order to be valued and validated.

Social media has become an intrinsic part of the lives of adolescent children. Being able to access an ever-increasing variety of apps has the potential to bring connection, community and information. However, we must also be aware that creating aspirational lifestyles available at the swipe of a screen creates a unique paradigm of pressure, comparison and self-judgement.

While parents and carers may have a sense of how education systems, for example, can influence how children grow up, they will never be able to understand being young with access to social media and how it shapes the behaviours of young people. This is an example of how vast the generation gap has become as a result of the introduction of technologies; a gap far greater than that of previous generations and their offspring. This discrepancy between their understanding as parents and their children being able to acquire the emotional literacy to be able to communicate their experience can be a source of misunderstanding, tension, confusion and pain.

Let me be clear, if young people are going through something, they do not need to be fixed, there is nothing wrong with them. They need love, support and understanding to work through their emotions and understand themselves better, finding safe and appropriate ways to express how they feel. These fundamental human skills are not enough of a part of how we educate our children but because of the way we live, they need to be. Integrative Breathwork and Strategic Emotional Empowerment give young people the tools to help them understand their emotions and default behavioural patterns, empowering them to make different decisions. Teenagers are not trying to make others' lives hard, they are desperately trying to figure themselves and their seemingly out of control emotions out. By equipping them with ways to tackle life head on and learning to read their emotions, we are making space for them to be the child that stole our hearts when they came into our lives.

EMBODYING BREATH TO MANAGE EMOTIONS

When you are feeling anxious or full of emotions that you don't know how to process, this exercise helps you to come out of your mind and into your body. The first step to self-regulation is awareness and taking in sensory information from both inside and outside your body. Connecting to your breath and being compassionate to your body helps you to be kinder to yourself and to others.

o Sit down on the floor or a bed. Pause to notice your body and breath. Relax your belly and take a few slower breaths into your belly.

o Move your shoulders and neck around and experience all the different sensations within your body.

o Massage your feet and toes and, breathing slowly, massage your calves and legs. Ask yourself – what am I feeling right now?

o Scan from your feet to your calves to your pelvis, torso and throat and notice any feelings.

o Massage your right arm slowly by gently squeezing the muscles from your shoulder to your elbow and down to your hands. Repeat on your left side. Be open to your feelings without trying to change, fix or deny them.

o Notice your thoughts. What story is your mind telling you? Is it a familiar story? Can you observe it with curiosity?

- Be kind and compassionate towards yourself and your feelings. Stay with your breath and notice how you feel. Keep your breath slow and mindful and rather than trying to push your emotions away, just sit with them.

Family isn't always blood

Family are the people in your life who are always there and have seen you at your worst and best and still want to have you in their lives. The ones who accept you for who you are. The ones who love and support you no matter what and build you up when you are down and vice versa. Whether you look forward to family gatherings or you get triggered by certain members, the breath is always a powerful tool to help manage those emotions when you get your buttons pushed or a throwaway comment makes you feel inadequate. It might be easy to take family for granted and as we move and grow dynamics change, but even if you can do nothing else, hugging, listening and being present help to keep us connected and supported.

HEART-TO-HEART BREATHING

A particular frequency of breath can be especially
restorative, triggering a 'relaxation response' in the brain
and body. When breathing slow, deep breaths with another
person, you set off a cascade of physiological responses
that induce a descent into a calm and unifying frequency
which can feel both soothing and relaxing.

o Sit comfortably, cross-legged, opposite each other.

o Place your right hand on your partner's heart centre
  (the middle of the chest) and your left hand on top of
  your partner's right hand.

o Close your eyes and breath in through your nose and
  out through your nose.

o Tune in to your breath and bring your focus from your mind
  to your heart space. Can you feel your heartbeat? How
  does your breath feel? Are your chest muscles relaxing?
  Can you feel expansion or openness, constriction? Do you
  notice vibrating, fluttering or peaceful feelings?

o Focus on the connection between your heart and
  your partner's hand and send love and warmth into your
  partner's heart, or you can gaze into each other's eyes
  (this can feel awkward, so just play with it).

o Notice if your breath begins to harmonise.

o When you feel ready, gently move your hands and bring
  your palms into prayer position and bow to each other
  to finish.

BACK-TO-BACK BREATHING

This is a simple exercise that many adults and children enjoy as children often like practising with another person rather than on their own. It is a safe and comfortable way of connecting with playfulness.

o Begin sitting up as tall as possible and back-to-back with your child, friend or family member.

o Take a few deep breaths and feel the support of your partner behind you, doing the same.

o Try not to push each other back or lean on one another; feel a mutual support between you. Notice each other's breath and back and ribs expanding.

o If you are enjoying this, play a bit more and move into 'bear on a rock' pose by one of you gently and slowly leaning forward while the other slowly leans back, opening their chest and expanding their ribs.

o Take a few breaths and then switch.

BREATHING WITH BABIES

It's never too young to begin breathing exercises. Naturally a newborn takes 30–50 breaths per minute; this can slow to 20 breaths while they sleep. Newborns can also take rapid breaths and then pause for up to 10 seconds at a time. All of this is very different from adult breathing patterns, which is why new parents might sometimes be alarmed. At six months, babies' breathing slows to around 20 breaths a minute. This is a really lovely exercise to practise with a newborn or baby that is a few months old.

o Sit in a comfortable chair. Hold the baby on your lap or a bit higher on your chest with the baby looking out.

o Lean back slightly and get comfortable. Breathe in and out until your breath and the baby's breath match. You can hold their belly lightly to feel their breath moving.

o This is really relaxing and can help with digestive issues or reflux in babies. You can very gently place your thumb or finger on their solar plexus as you breathe and the baby breathes.

EXERCISES FOR LITTLE BREATHERS

The following exercises are for younger children to understand how they can boost their own energy and connect to their senses.

Eye-palming breath

o Heartily rub the palms of your hands together until they begin to feel warm.

o Close your eyes and place your palms gently over your eyes. Feel the warmth and cocoon-like feeling enveloping your eyes. Breathe a little deeper.

o With the palms still over your eyes, gently open them letting light filter through.

o As your eyes adjust to the light, continue breathing softly and then bring your hands back down to rest on your thighs or knees.

Making an energy ball

This is a fun way to feel energy and practise how to focus.

o Take a few deep breaths into the belly. Bring the hands together and begin to rub your palms vigorously until your hands feel warm.

o Stop and imagine that in between the hands is a ball of energy.

o As you take a deep breath in and out the light is growing and expanding filling the hands with energy.

o Gently move the palms of the hands apart on the inhale, slowly pulling them away from each other.

o On the exhale, slowly push your hands back together.

o Often you feel that your palms act like two magnets pushing each other away.

o Continue expanding your energy ball as you breathe in and squeezing it together as you breathe out, keeping the rest of your body as still as you can.

o Use the inhale and exhale to match the length of the expanding and contracting so it should take the entire length of your inhalation to bring your hands apart.

o It should also take the entire length of your exhalation to push them back together.

o Then see if you can expand the ball and roll around it while moving your hands. Expanding and contracting the ball.

o When they have finished the exercise, ask the child what they felt and if the energy ball felt strong or if they could feel just a little heat or vibration. If your child (or you) is having trouble feeling the energy in their hands, don't worry! When we aren't used to feeling something it can take a little bit of time to find it.

Hissing breath

Teaching children to connect to their exhale helps them learn to how to slow themselves down, mentally and physically. Extending the exhale will allow kids to slow down their inner thoughts.

- Breathe in through your nose – a long, deep inhale.

- Exhale out through your mouth with a hissing sound, slow and long.

Lion breath

This will help ground and settle children. It's wonderful for shifting their focus or for a more reflective time such as storytime or any creative activity.

- Sit in a cross-legged position or with your knees tucked underneath you.

- Inhale through your nose, pause; exhale through your nose, pause.

- Breathe in for a count of three or four, pause for a count of one or two; breath out for a count of three or four, pause for a count of one or two. Repeat a few times.

- Place the palms of your hands on the floor in front of you.

- Inhale and then open your mouth and stick out your tongue, rest it on your lower lip and exhale with a roar.

- Repeat 3–4 times.

Bunny breath

Invite children to pretend to be rabbits, sniffing the air for carrots to eat or a safe space to burrow. You can use this exercise when children are upset and can't find their breath, as it will help them connect to their exhale, so that they breathe instead of spinning out of control. It is also good for focus and energising.

o Take three quick sniffs in through your nose and one long exhale out through the nose.

Cool down breath

When energy is high and it's time to cool down, practise this cooling breath – it's a bit like creating your own air conditioning system.

o Find a comfortable seated position with a straight spine. Relax your shoulders.

o Curl the edges of your tongue together like a straw, if your tongue doesn't curl make a little round straw with your lips.

o Take a deep breath in through your straw. Hold your breath for a second, then gently breathe out through your mouth. Repeat for a few rounds.

BREATHING WITH THE ELDERLY

You can do this exercise with grandparents or elderly relatives when they are not very mobile. The soothing connection of touch is bonding for both participants. If your grandparent or elderly relative is bed-bound or has a favourite chair, pull up a chair next to them. This can help with breathlessness and tightness in the chest and invoke feelings of love in the heart and lightness in the body. It's important to ask them not to force the breath or take deep breaths. This is a gentle connecting exercise that is subtle as well as comforting and peaceful.

- Place your hand gently on their belly and ask them to feel your hand on their belly and to gently breathe into it.

- Stay present with their breath and present with your breath. Not trying to control the timing, depth or rhythm of the breath.

- You can both close your eyes if that feels comfortable and maybe play some relaxing music, or simply be in the silence.

- Bring your hand to the middle of their chest and gently rest your hand there. Encourage them to gently breathe into your hand and feel its warmth on their chest.

- If there is any tightness in their chest, you can gently place your second and third finger under the clavicle (collarbone) and just stay present with their breath. Encourage them to breathe gently into their belly.

- Under the clavicle you will find two little pockets that dip in either side. Place your thumb and index finger on the pockets gently and just stay present with the breath. In Chinese medicine these little pockets are said to be like a little well where we store the tears we haven't expressed. Simply allow the space for them to breathe and feel into here.

CYCLES

THE CYCLES OF LIFE

The cycles of nature teach us about rhythms, including the circadian rhythm of day to night, balance, letting go and reciprocity. By being more in tune with the seasons, cycles of the moon and your own body's cycles, you can bring harmony and balance into your life and the world around you. This last year the world has been turned on its axis by the coronavirus pandemic and writing this book has not been a linear process. I listened to my body and worked with my own cycles and the seasons, not pushing myself when I felt blocked or tired and allowing myself to be in the flow. It's not always easy when there are deadlines and choosing to work in this way takes a lot of trust. Needless to say, I was late on delivery but I feel this book is richer for it.

Cycles remind us to be aware of our surroundings and others, to consider our actions, to understand that we are part of a larger whole and every thought, action and reaction has a ripple effect. Cycles teach us about nurturing, resting, caring for the planet and ourselves. They teach us about life, learning and growing. Nature doesn't resist force but moves gracefully, breathing through it all while remaining malleable. Trees and plants root firmly in the ground but still sway with the wind, surrendering to the rhythms of life without resistance. Life doesn't have to be linear or mapped out and often you'll find that when you're dancing to its rhythms rather than trying to push through, it feels like less of a battle.

> 'Life is a series of natural and spontaneous changes. Don't resist them – that only creates sorrow. Let reality be reality. Let things flow naturally forward in whatever way they like.' Lao Tzu

Masculine and feminine cycles

There is a lot of generalisation of women's and men's cycles and much is still not fully researched. It is said that the working day is structured around studies which show men's twenty-four-hour testosterone cycle peaks in the morning and retreats back to the metaphorical cave in the evening. Most men have about ten times more testosterone than women, so their hormone cycle primarily revolves around how their testosterone affects them.

A man does produce oestrogen and progesterone like a woman, but in much smaller amounts. The way we talk about the menstrual cycle can be isolating for people who don't identify with female labels or language. It's important to note that trans men and non-binary people also get periods and that not all women menstruate. As we grow in an ever-changing world we need to be more open to accepting that we are all individual and, like nature, our cycles ever evolving.

Nurturing both the masculine and feminine is essential in order to achieve balance. Are you running too much masculine energy or a little too wrapped up in your feminine energy? And what does that mean? In Chinese medicine, yang refers to masculine energy and yin to feminine; they both exist within every one of us, regardless of our sex and gender. When in opposition they struggle against each other. When there is a healthy interdependence, they define each other. The masculine works in a more linear way whereas the feminine is more flowing and fluid. Our world is currently in masculine overdrive, pushing forwards with no regard for consequences and an overriding domination and reckless overuse of the Earth's resources for personal or industrial gain. We've found ourselves in a time of excessive masculinity, which has led to a culture of overachievement and overconsumption where we feel overworked and depleted. When in balance, the masculine offers structure, practicality, logic, discipline and organisation. When the masculine is allowed its true expression, it keeps us on track with our vision and goals. Where the masculine focuses on growth and production, the feminine brings us into alignment and embodiment. Flowing and spiralling intuitively in the midst of creation. Feminine cultivates a gentle authority of acceptance, emotional expression and pleasure. The feminine brings us into our feeling, senses and our ever-changing bodies.

BUTTERFLY POSE BREATH

This simple breathing exercise helps restore balance to the body and mind. This restorative stretch relieves tension in your inner thighs, groin and knees.

o Find a comfortable, quiet space and allow yourself ten minutes to do this.

o Lie down with a pillow beneath your head. Bend your knees and bring the soles of your feet together. Gently let your legs flop out to the sides (resting thighs on cushions or bolsters if you need to). Relax your belly and tune in to your breath.

o Place your hands on your belly and as you inhale feel your belly rise, as you exhale feel it go down. Allow the exhale to be relaxed.

o Simply follow your breath as it enters and leaves your body. Allow it to be effortless and relaxed.

o Inhale and focus on your left side. As you breathe, visualise your breath moving along your left side.

o With the flow of the inhale and exhale, allow your focus to travel from your left foot up to your left shoulder. Continue until you feel this side is more spacious and flowing.

o Shift your focus to your right side. Inhale through your right shoulder and down into the right side of your body. Each inhale has a cooling and calming effect and the exhale gently releases any tension.

○ Continue alternating your focus between your left and
  right sides until you feel an evenness of energy between
  both sides.

○ With each breath use the affirmations 'I am in perfect
  balance and harmony' and 'I surrender and let go'.
  Breathe and feel yourself gently letting go.

TAKE TIME TO REFLECT AND WRITE

Here are some questions to help you figure out how your work and life could flow more closely with cycles and the seasons:

o Do you feel you have a work/life balance? Are there any patterns you notice around this?

o Do you find it hard to switch off? Are you aware of when you may be reaching burnout or do you push on through it? What activity allows you to switch off?

o What are the signs of sacrifice in your life or working against your own natural rhythms?

o How can nature teach you to reset and rewire to be more productive in your working hours? How can you help yourself switch off when work becomes stressful or an unhealthy factor in your identity?

o How would you envisage a future to manage work/ life balance?

o Are there times when you find you are more productive in the year or month? Do you find there are days or months where you are more creative or organised?

o When do you feel your body needs the most rest and when does it have the most energy?

Menstruation and menopause

Working with your menstrual/hormonal cycle means
making space to know when you are fragile and need to
push back a little, when your creativity is flowing, when
your voice is strong, when you want solitude and when you
feel social. These gentle exercises combine movement,
stretches and your breath to help reduce stress and
anxiety, digestive or hormonal bloating. They also help
relax the nervous system and restore balance.

HAPPY BABY

This is a really gentle stretch for the hips and lower back while massaging the stomach.

o Lie on your back and bring your knees into your chest. Take hold of the ball of each foot (if you can't reach that far, hold your ankles or calves).

o Open your legs wide, keeping the knees close to the body but extending the heels towards the sky and breathe deeply. You can stay still here for 30 seconds or gently rock from side to side to make the move more active.

WIND RELEASE POSE

Also known as *pavanamuktasana* which, roughly translated from Sanskrit, means 'wind-removing pose'. This practice is used in yoga and is great for when digestion or trapped wind is causing bloating.

o Lie on your back with your legs extended straight and your arms by your sides.

o Hug one leg in towards your chest with both arms.

o Slightly turn the leg out so that your knee comes towards your shoulder. Point the toe of the leg that's extended to stretch the front of your hip. Hold for 15 seconds.

o Repeat on the opposite side.

SUPINE SPINAL TWIST

Supine spinal twist pose, also referred to as reclined spinal twist, is a simple and effective beginner's yoga pose. This exercise stretches the glutes, chest, and obliques. Because of the chest stretch, it is considered a heart opener. It improves spinal mobility and can aid digestion. It is a relaxing pose at the end of a yoga session. In everyday life, your posture will benefit from this antidote to sitting and hunching over work.

o Lie on your back and hug one knee in towards your chest.

o With your opposite hand, pull the leg across the body and down towards the floor. Try to get your knee to touch the ground without lifting your shoulder too far off the ground. Hold for 15 seconds.

o Repeat on the opposite side. Remember to breathe throughout!

Lunar Cycles

The moon is our closest celestial neighbour and has a powerful influence on every living thing on the planet, including the ocean and the seasons – exerting two and a half times the gravitational pull of the sun. Have you ever found you can't sleep or feel overly emotional, exhausted or filled with the need to make big changes and start something completely new for no reason? Chances are that you are tuning into the energetic cycles of the moon without knowing it. We can learn a lot from the moon and its cycles, and in turn tune in to its energies to help us to continue flowing with the cycles of life. Using the moon's energy to let go helps you to create space for new beginnings and amazing opportunities, continue growing and moving forwards.

PAULA'S MOON RITUAL

For this chapter I asked my dear friend and master teacher in astrology, meditation and ritual, Paula Shaw to share her wisdom. She has guided me through many a cycle in my life.

When in your life do you actually give yourself permission to just let go? When was the last time you decided you were done with something? True letting go is a moment of taking back power from events and people in your life that are holding you back, pulling you down or creating negative repetitive loops.

Until you decide to let go, you are left spinning on repeat. You feel miserable, stuck and totally trapped and confused! Performing a ritual is a potent way to decide how you feel about your life and to take action on those decisions. Ritual helps you take back the reins of your life, grow in confidence and gain a stronger sense of self-mastery. When you know what the fundamentals of ritual practices are, you will see how much of what you already do is ritual. By definition, a ritual is a moment where you engage in an act where the meaning and purpose of the act is greater than the act itself. A great example is cleaning your home. The act of cleaning your home becomes a ritual when you understand the greater purpose and meaning of why you are doing it. When you tune into why you are cleaning, you get to the heart of the greater purpose, which for many of us is about creating a harmonious space for ourselves and our loved ones. When you connect to this higher value, the act of cleaning becomes a sacred ritual. Your entire life can be a ritual. The more you let go of the past, of fear and of pain, the more you relax and connect with your personal wisdom and a greater meaning for your life is revealed. This greater meaning gives you the courage and power to steer your life towards what really matters to you.

Many cultures work with the phases of the moon to empower their lives, to mark time, to gather, to connect with the natural cycles of nature and to remember what is sacred. Traditionally the full moon is the time to let go, release and purify. Full moons are a time of amplification where everything is heightened, especially emotions, and you can more easily access what is disturbing you and is ready to be released. I want to share with you a simple letting go ritual that you can do on your own.

FULL MOON EXERCISE

The full moon is the ideal time for completion and letting go, so at the next full moon, find a quiet space for this exercise.

○ Grab some paper, a pen, a candle, some incense and anything else that helps you to connect with what you are feeling.

○ Take time feeling what you are ready to let go of. Listen to what is going on internally. We all know what we are holding on to or what is repeating in our lives, but most of us are too busy to listen. Really listen and write down what is coming up, feel it pour on to the paper.

○ Burn what you have written over the candle as a gesture of fully letting it go. Sometimes you may feel you have let go instantly and sometimes you may work with this ritual multiple times as you build up your internal strength to that tipping point where it all just falls away.

○ Know that as you let go of what doesn't matter, what truly matters is revealed to you and your life then fills up with richness of meaning and connection to what is truly sacred to you.

○ When practising this exercise, you can also work with your breath. In everyday life we never fully exhale and so are always holding on to something. Inhale fully, then exhale until you think there is nothing left and then exhale more and more to really feel the effects of fully letting go. Hold your breath at the end of exhale until the inhale comes in naturally on its own. Visualise the light of the moon shining down on you and breathe in that light to allow release anywhere it's needed physically, emotionally or mentally.

The seasons

Being here right now is a gift; to be alive and in harmony with nature and all the elements can be a spiritual experience, so let nature be your church and each breath a prayer. To regain balance, take time to reflect, study and remember how we used to work with cycles and ritual, particularly those of the seasons.

From autumn to winter the Earth breathes in and draws energy downwards, nourishing the soil and roots. Over the spring and summer the Earth breathes out, sending energy into plants and working with the rhythms of the sun and the moon. As winter sets in, we can tune in to the cycle that brings in stillness and space to reflect and retreat. In summer we can celebrate the longer days, warmth and the manifestations of nature bringing life into fruition.

BREATHING WITH THE ELEMENTS

Use this exercise as an energy transfer, letting go of anything heavy and offering it to the ground, then visualising that energy being transformed into the Earth like compost and coming back to you as vibrant, effervescent light. This exercise connects you to the elements around and inside you: earth, air, water and fire.

o Go outside and find your favourite tree, park, space in your garden, stream or water. Stand or sit on the ground. Take a few breaths and notice the sounds and temperature around you.

o Imagine you have roots coming from your feet growing into the ground, connecting you to the Earth beneath you. Take a deep breath in and out and feel your connection to the ground beneath you. As you breathe in, feel the energy of the Earth coming up through you. Exhale and send anything down to the Earth that no longer serves you, letting go of any heaviness. As you inhale, feel the transformed energy travelling up into your body while honouring this exchange between you and the Earth.

o Close your eyes and breathe into the fire within you, deep in your core, that burns inside, this light ignites more with each breath. Visualise the heat of the sun on your skin and as you breathe feel the sun's warmth all over your body.

o Inhale and exhale and connect to the water inside you, your blood that carries nutrients to your cells and the water around you that keeps you cleansed and hydrated. Breathe in and breathe out and connect to the flow within you and ask the spirit of water to help your flow.

o Breathe in and out and connect to the air you breathe. Inhale, giving thanks to the air that keeps you alive and the oxygen that feeds your cells. Giving gratitude to the air you breathe, the trees and plants that exchange the gases, the water that keeps all plants and living creatures alive and the sun that gives light to all life.

SUN MEDITATION

This is a balancing way to begin your day. If you're not able to soak up the sun because it's winter or a rainy day, try to visualise its golden rays. If the sun is shining, focus on its light infiltrating and charging every cell of your body, healing and rejuvenating you.

Practise this sitting or lying down, indoors or outdoors. For maximum benefit, I recommend sitting up.

o Close your eyes, tune in to your breath and connect to the ground beneath you. Feel your sitting bones on the ground and keep your spine straight.

o Breathe in and out, deeply down into your belly. Place your hands on your belly and visualise a glowing ball of fire or light within your core. As you inhale, this light expands and as you exhale it contracts.

o Visualise a thread coming from the ball of light down to the base of your spine and into the Earth. The thread travels through the Earth until it reaches its core of burning-hot magma. Feel the connection of the sun to the Earth and the sun inside you and breathe into this as you visualise this connection charging you up.

o Bring your focus back to the thread and travel back up to the ball of light within you, then up your spine, through your head, all the way up to the sun in the sky.

o As you breathe in and out, feel your breath moving through you and visualise the connection between the sun below (Earth's core), the sun (ball of light) inside your core and the sun in the sky, powering you with warmth and light.

o Feel this cosmic energy travelling back from the sun in the sky, down through the top of your head, into your belly and down into the Earth's core. Feel the powerful connection of the three suns inside, below and above. Now breathe in and take this feeling of warmth and light out into your day, keeping you fully charged and ready to go wherever the breath decides to take you.

EXERCISE INDEX

This index is here to help you dip in and out and find
what you need when you need it. It covers my favourite
exercises from the book.

On The Go
Perfect for when you are out and about.

At Home Retreat
These are for when you have more time and want to
create a little sanctuary for yourself.

At work

These are perfect for the work environment. They will help you focus, improve productivity and boost confidence.

For the Commute (not when driving!)

For those still moments when going from A to B.

Soothing Nervous Energy

Energy Boost

In Nature

Bedtime

Balance
Exercises to help you find emotional balance day-to-day.

Health

ACKNOWLEDGEMENTS

I feel deeply grateful for the opportunity to write another book on a subject that I am incredibly passionate about. A huge thank you to all-round wonderful human being Fearne Cotton for asking me to share my knowledge with Happy Place Books. It's such an honour to do this with you and the brilliant Happy Place crew. You are a beacon of light and inspiration and bring so much joy and hope to others.

A huge thank you to the brilliantly innovate team at Penguin. You are all a breath of fresh air to work with and so creative. Thank you for giving me freedom, extra time and allowing me to share my vision and my voice – Laura Higginson, Samantha Crisp, Vicky Orchard – you all rock.

Thank you to Jordan McGarry for all the wisdom and edits for my initial vision of *Let It Go* and your time and chats and general awesomeness. Also thank you to Rebecca Hull for reading every page before I had to let it go, holding my hand and reminding me to breathe. Thank you to Valeria Huerta and Amanda Harris for being on this journey with me and for all that you do.

Enormous gratitude to the courageous and inspiring contributors who generously agreed to share their stories and words of wisdom for *Let It Go*. What you have shared is so important and I know will help so many who will resonate with your words. Mark Whittle, Rebecca Hull, Ella Oliver, Jessica Horn, Michele Barocchi, Bea Adamson, Paula Shaw, Abbie Eastwood, Ria Ingleby, I don't think I can thank you all enough. I am in total awe of you all which I why I wanted so much for you to be a part of this book.

My beautiful son, Louis, my greatest teacher of all who is wise beyond years and will always pull me up for not being present! Of all the teachers I've had over the years I've learnt the most from you. I am so proud to be your mum and thank you for your understanding and patience when I had to work into weekends and nights. You are my world and my inspiration and may the breath give you wings to be whoever you wish to be in this life. Massive thank you to Tom for taking on the large majority of home schooling so I could write and giving Louis the most magical few months of lock down.

My darling mum for bearing with me on the walks in the woods when all I can talk about is the book and deadlines and always being there for me through the highs and the lows. Thank you to all my incredible friends who've been there at the end of the line to keep me sane, make me laugh and unpack the route towards a balanced and sustainable world! Thank you to all my clients who continue to teach me every day.

Biggest thank you to the greatest mother of all, Nature. When I've been lost for words and need space, I come to you, when my mind is overwhelmed and I have found it hard to process emotions that have come up in these uncertain times you have been there to ground and calm me. I feel so grateful to be able to sit by the stream and with the trees and just breathe and listen. In this mutual exchange of air, you have been the wisdom I needed to help me remember who I am and how sacred every breath and life is.

The breath for me is always the star of the show and every day I am grateful to be able to breathe. Even in the darkest of times we can find the brightest of lights. The breath is always there to guide us through and love is always the way. It's up to us to choose that. Just remember, we are all connected in this ocean of air together. It's the breath that connects us all. PEACE.

FURTHER READING

Here are some of my favourite go-tos for you to consider . . .

Lisa Feldman Barrett, How Emotions Are Made: The Secret Life of the Brain (Pan, 2018).

Donna Fahri, The Breathing Book: Vitality and Good Health Through Essential Breath Work (Holt (Henry) & Co, U.S., 1996).

Sue Gerhardt, Why Love Matters: How Affection Shapes a Baby's Brain (Routledge, 2014).

Daniel Goleman, Emotional Intelligence: Why it Can Matter More Than IQ (Bloomsbury Publishing, 1996).

Daniel Goleman & Richard J. Davidson, The Science of Meditation: How to Change Your Brain, Mind and Body (Penguin Life, 2018).

Stephen Grosz, The Examined Life: How We Lose and Find Ourselves (Vintage, 2014).

Thich Nhat Hanh, Teachings on Love (Full Circle Publishing Ltd, 2007).

Anodea Judith, Eastern Body, Western Mind: Psychology and the Chakra System as a Path to the Self (Potter/Ten Speed/Harmony/Rodale, 2004).

Bessel van der Kolk, The Body Keeps the Score: Mind, Brain and Body in the Transformation of Trauma (Penguin, 2015).

Peter A. Levine, Waking The Tiger: Healing Trauma: The Innate Capacity to Transform Overwhelming Experiences (North Atlantic Books, U.S., 1977).

Joanna Macy, Widening Circles: A Memoir (New Catalyst Books, 2007).

Patrick McKeown, The Oxygen Advantage: Simple, Scientifically Proven Breathing Techniques to Help You Become Healthier, Slimmer, Faster and Fitter (William Morrow & Company, 2016).

Marlo Morgan, Mutant Message Down Under: A Woman's Journey into Dreamtime Australia (Thorsons, 1994).

James Nestor, Breath: The New Science of a Lost Art (Penguin Life, 2020).

Yogi Ramacharaka, Science of Breath (Watchmaker Publishing, 2011).

Swami Saradananda, The Power Of Breath: Yoga Breathing for Inner Balance, Health and Harmony (Watkins Publishing, 2017).

Michael A. Singer, The Untethered Soul: The Journey Beyond Yourself (New Harbinger Publications, 2007).

Max Strom, A Life Worth Breathing: A Yoga Master's Handbook of Strength, Grace and Healing (Skyhorse Publishing, 2012).

Alberto Villoldo, One Spirit Medicine: Ancient Ways to Ultimate Wellness (Hay House, 2015).

Neale Donald Walsch, Conversations With God, Book 1: An Uncommon Dialogue (Hodder & Stoughton, 1997).

Happy Place Books, an imprint of Ebury Publishing,

20 Vauxhall Bridge Road,
London SW1V 2SA

Happy Place Books is part of the Penguin Random House group of companies
whose addresses can be found at global.penguinrandomhouse.com

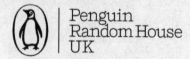

Penguin
Random House
UK

Text Copyright © Rebecca Dennis

Rebecca Dennis has asserted her right to be identified as the author of this
Work in accordance with the Copyright, Designs and Patents Act 1988

First published by Happy Place Books in 2021
This paperback edition published in 2022

www.penguin.co.uk

A CIP catalogue record for this book is available from the British Library

ISBN 9781529909739

Text Design Seagull Design
Cover Design by Heike Schüssler
Illustrations by Pirrip Press
Printed and bound in Great Britain by Clays Ltd, Elcograf S.p.A.

The authorised representative in the EEA is Penguin Random House Ireland,
Morrison Chambers, 32 Nassau Street, Dublin D02 YH68